PEPTIDES

FOR BIOHACKERS

The Ultimate Guide to Anti-Aging, Fat Loss, Muscle
Recovery, Sleep Optimization, and Peak Vitality

Oliver Wilson

TABLE OF CONTENTS

PREFACE

Welcome to Peptides for Biohackers: The Ultimate Guide to Anti-Aging, Fat Loss, Muscle Recovery, Sleep Optimization, and Peak Vitality. This book is your gateway into the powerful and ever-expanding world of peptides—designed specifically for high achievers and health-focused individuals seeking to unlock greater vitality through science-backed methods.

If you're reading this, you likely thrive on optimization. You monitor your sleep, track your HRV, fine-tune your workouts, and pursue peak physical and mental performance. You might be an entrepreneur, a fitness enthusiast, or a wellness professional committed to staying ahead of the curve.

Peptides represent one of the most promising frontiers in biohacking. But with the explosion of information—often fragmented, overly technical, or contradictory—it's easy to feel lost. This guide was created to bring clarity. It cuts through the noise to offer a precise, well-structured, and user-friendly roadmap to peptide use.

This book blends cutting-edge research with practical application. You'll explore the science behind peptides, discover their potential for anti-aging, fat loss, muscle repair, cognitive enhancement, and sleep regulation, and learn how to create protocols tailored to your individual goals.

The insights here are built on scientific literature, interviews with experts, and real-life case studies. But while the foundation is solid, the landscape continues to evolve. New compounds are emerging. Protocols are being refined. What you'll find in these pages is a strong starting point—an up-to-date framework designed to adapt alongside your own experimentation and growth.

Peptides are not standalone fixes. They are tools—powerful, yes, but most effective when integrated into a broader lifestyle of smart nutrition, consistent exercise, quality sleep, and mindful living. Your progress will depend not only on the compounds you choose, but also on how you support them with daily habits.

My hope is that this book equips you with both knowledge and direction. Whether you're exploring peptides for the first time or refining your current stack, you'll find the structure and insight needed to advance your practice with confidence and clarity.

Welcome to Peptides for Biohackers.

— Oliver Wilson

INTRODUCTION

What Are Peptides and Why They Matter in Biohacking

Peptides are short chains of amino acids—the same fundamental units that build proteins, but on a much smaller scale. While proteins are composed of more than 50 amino acids, peptides range from just two to fifty. This seemingly minor difference in size gives peptides unique biological advantages.

Their compact structure allows them to cross physiological barriers like the skin, the gut lining, and even the blood-brain barrier. Once inside the body, they act as precise messengers, delivering instructions to cells and triggering targeted biological responses.

Unlike proteins, which serve structural or enzymatic functions, peptides often serve as signaling molecules. They bind to specific receptors and activate precise cellular functions—stimulating growth hormone, accelerating tissue repair, modulating inflammation, and influencing neurochemical balance, among many other effects.

This signaling ability makes peptides especially valuable for biohackers. With the right peptide, you can influence the body's internal messaging systems to enhance muscle recovery, improve sleep quality, increase fat metabolism, or support cellular regeneration.

For example, a peptide that boosts growth hormone levels can aid in muscle development and fat loss. Another might stimulate the production of melatonin to support circadian rhythm regulation and better sleep. Others promote wound healing, reduce oxidative stress, or enhance cognitive performance. Each peptide offers a specific and controllable biological input.

The potential applications are broad. Whether you're targeting aesthetic improvements like skin rejuvenation, systemic goals like improved immune resilience, or deeper anti-aging objectives like DNA repair, peptides offer tools with measurable effects and low systemic burden.

Although peptides are gaining traction among performance enthusiasts, they also hold significant promise in clinical medicine. Because of their selectivity and safety profile, peptides are being explored as therapeutic agents for conditions ranging from inflammatory diseases to neurodegeneration, cardiovascular dysfunction, and even cancer.

Many of today's most popular peptides were first developed for medical purposes. BPC-157, now favored by athletes and biohackers for its regenerative and anti-inflammatory properties, originated in gastrointestinal research. Its ability to accelerate healing is now applied far beyond its original therapeutic target.

Despite the excitement, it's crucial to approach peptides with a scientific mindset. The field is still young, and although many peptides show great promise, clinical validation is ongoing. Misuse, poor sourcing, or inadequate dosing can reduce efficacy or cause unintended effects. Careful planning, ongoing monitoring, and ideally guidance from an experienced provider are essential for safe and effective use.

Peptides offer direct access to some of the body's most powerful biological systems. For biohackers seeking strategic interventions to enhance performance, slow aging, and recover faster, they represent a frontier rich with opportunity.

This guide is built to help you understand how peptides work, what they can do, and how to use them responsibly to support your health goals. Whether you're exploring peptides for the first time or optimizing a well-established protocol, the tools and knowledge are here.

The Rise of Peptide Therapy in Modern Health Optimization

Peptide therapy has roots extending back to the early 20th century. The discovery of insulin in the 1920s marked the first major milestone in medical peptide application. Since then, peptides have steadily gained relevance, but it is only in the last two decades that their full potential in health optimization has begun to emerge.

Several key factors have driven this resurgence. One is the deepening understanding of how peptides function within the body. As scientific insight into cellular communication has advanced, so too has recognition of peptides as precise biological messengers capable of directing highly specific responses—stimulating tissue repair, modulating hormones, reducing inflammation, and more.

At the same time, technological advancements have transformed how peptides are made and applied. Laboratory synthesis has enabled the creation of custom peptides designed for targeted effects. This capability has given rise to a broad spectrum of therapeutic options, each tailored to influence distinct physiological systems with minimal side effects.

The rise of biohacking has also played a central role. As more people adopt a proactive, data-driven approach to personal health, the demand for tools that offer measurable benefits with high specificity has grown. Peptides align with this ethos. They can be personalized, combined, and cycled to support unique goals—ranging from longevity to athletic performance.

Results have fueled interest further. Reports of improved muscle growth, accelerated fat loss, deeper sleep, sharper cognition, and faster recovery continue to mount. Although much of the scientific literature is still developing, real-world experiences have validated many of these effects. Enthusiasts and clinicians alike are documenting impressive outcomes.

Nevertheless, this growing field is not without challenges. Regulatory inconsistencies, limited long-term research, and variations in product quality can create barriers to safe and effective use. Additionally, access to knowledgeable professionals remains uneven, and misinformation is common in unregulated spaces.

Despite these concerns, the trajectory of peptide therapy is promising. Innovations in biotechnology continue to yield more refined compounds with improved bioavailability and fewer side effects. As research catches up with practice, evidence-based guidelines will become more accessible, helping users integrate peptides more responsibly.

More broadly, peptide therapy reflects a fundamental shift in health optimization. It's not just about adding a new tool—it represents a move toward precision interventions, grounded in biology and tailored to the individual. This direction resonates with a growing recognition that effective health strategies must be personal, adaptable, and backed by both data and clinical insight.

Peptides are not a universal solution, but they are a versatile and impactful addition to a well-designed protocol. When used with intention, informed planning, and appropriate monitoring, they offer unique leverage in the pursuit of sustained wellness, performance, and vitality.

This evolving field continues to invite curiosity and experimentation, especially for those who view health as an active pursuit. Peptide therapy stands at the crossroads of science and self-mastery, offering a path to targeted, high-impact outcomes grounded in biological intelligence.

How to Use This Book for Safe, Strategic Results

This book is structured to serve as both a reference and a roadmap—designed to guide you through the science and application of peptides with clarity and precision. Whether you're exploring peptides for the first time or refining a long-standing regimen, this resource will help you make informed, effective decisions tailored to your health goals.

The opening chapters establish the scientific foundation. Here, you'll gain a clear understanding of what peptides are, how they work, and why they matter in the context of health optimization. This section is essential for building the conceptual framework you'll rely on as you explore specific use cases later.

Subsequent chapters focus on targeted applications—muscle development, fat reduction, sleep enhancement, cognitive support, skin health, and more. Each section identifies relevant peptides, explains their mechanisms of action, and outlines practical guidance for implementation. Dosing protocols, administration methods, and expected outcomes are all addressed with a focus on usability and safety.

Beyond isolated compounds, the book emphasizes how to develop a strategic peptide protocol. You'll learn how to align peptide selection with your goals, how to combine compounds for synergistic effects, and how to manage timing and cycling for sustainable benefits. The approach is modular—flexible enough to accommodate individual differences while grounded in biological logic.

A core principle of this guide is personalization. Health optimization must be tailored. What works for one individual may be ineffective or counterproductive for another. This book offers a toolkit of options and frameworks to help you customize your protocol based on your physiology, lifestyle, and objectives.

Safety is prioritized throughout. Responsible peptide use begins with sourcing—understanding where and how to obtain quality compounds. It continues with proper storage, preparation, and administration. Risks and potential side effects are addressed with actionable strategies to reduce harm and improve outcomes.

This is a book meant to evolve with you. As your goals shift, as new research emerges, and as you gain experience, you'll find value in returning to these chapters. It's a reference that supports long-term engagement with the peptide landscape.

More than a collection of information, this book is designed to empower you with strategic insight. Peptides are powerful tools—but their effectiveness depends on how they're used. With the right understanding, you can unlock significant gains in performance, recovery, vitality, and longevity.

Approach this material with intention. Study the science, apply the strategies, and monitor the results. Make adjustments as needed, guided by data and experience. This isn't about shortcuts—it's about intelligent, sustained self-optimization.

The knowledge is here. The structure is in place. The results will come from how you engage with it.

CHAPTER 1
PEPTIDES 101
– WHAT YOU NEED TO KNOW

The Science Behind Peptides

Peptides are short chains of amino acids, the fundamental components of all proteins. While proteins are composed of 50 or more amino acids, peptides consist of just two to fifty, granting them unique biological advantages. Their compact structure allows them to cross cellular barriers, including the skin, the intestinal lining, and even the blood-brain barrier. This gives peptides the ability to act directly on specific tissues and organs with remarkable precision.

What sets peptides apart from proteins is their role as signaling molecules. Once a peptide binds to a cell receptor, it activates a cascade of intracellular processes—essentially instructing the cell to perform a particular function. These functions can include stimulating growth hormone production, reducing inflammation, initiating tissue repair, or regulating metabolic activity.

This signaling capability is the foundation of peptide therapy. By selectively introducing peptides into the body, we can engage with its internal communication systems and enhance specific biological responses. For those focused on performance, recovery, and longevity, this opens the door to targeted interventions with measurable outcomes.

Many peptides already exist within the body. Insulin, for example, is a peptide that regulates blood glucose by signaling cells to absorb sugar from the bloodstream. Oxytocin promotes bonding and trust by acting on receptors in the brain. These examples illustrate how vital peptides are in orchestrating everyday physiological functions.

In addition to those naturally produced by the body, researchers have developed synthetic peptides that replicate or enhance natural signals. These lab-created compounds can be tailored to influence precise pathways—supporting goals like muscle development, fat metabolism, immune support, cognitive enhancement, and more.

Peptide levels tend to decline with age, contributing to slower recovery, reduced metabolic efficiency, and diminished hormonal balance. Supplementing with carefully selected peptides may help restore these signaling patterns and slow age-related decline.

However, because peptides are biologically active, their use requires care. Improper selection, dosing, or sourcing can result in unintended consequences. Responsible use should always involve a foundation of scientific understanding, quality sourcing, and ideally professional oversight.

Regulatory status varies widely. Some peptides are readily available as research compounds or dietary aids, while others are restricted to clinical settings. Legal considerations must be taken into account before beginning any peptide protocol, and sourcing should be transparent and verifiable.

Peptides represent a powerful interface between science and self-optimization. Their precision, versatility, and broad spectrum of effects make them an invaluable tool in the modern biohacker's toolkit. But like all potent technologies, they demand respect, careful planning, and a commitment to evidence-based use.

Understanding how peptides function—and how to use them strategically—forms the essential groundwork for deeper exploration.

How They Differ from Hormones and Proteins

To fully grasp the potential of peptides, it's essential to distinguish them from two related biological molecules: proteins and hormones. While all three play critical roles in maintaining health and regulating physiology, they differ significantly in structure, function, and application.

Peptides are composed of amino acids, just like proteins. The distinction lies in size. Proteins are long, complex chains containing more than fifty amino acids, often folded into intricate three-dimensional structures. Peptides, by contrast, are shorter sequences—typically ranging from two to fifty amino acids.

This structural simplicity gives peptides several unique advantages. Due to their smaller size, they can cross biological barriers such as the intestinal lining, the skin, and even the blood-brain barrier. Proteins, being larger and more complex, generally cannot. Their effects are often localized to the cells where they're produced or require specific transport mechanisms to act elsewhere.

Hormones function as messengers—chemical signals released by glands that travel through the bloodstream to influence distant organs. They regulate critical functions such as metabolism, growth, reproduction, and mood. Many hormones are peptides themselves. Examples include insulin, which manages glucose uptake; glucagon, which raises blood sugar; and growth hormone-releasing hormone (GHRH), which stimulates the release of growth hormone.

However, not all hormones are peptides. Steroid hormones—like cortisol, estrogen, and testosterone—are derived from cholesterol, not amino acids. This fundamental difference affects their solubility, transport, and receptor interactions. Peptide hormones are water-soluble and typically act on surface receptors, while steroid hormones are lipid-soluble and pass directly into cells to bind intracellular receptors.

Another distinction lies in origin. Proteins and natural hormones are synthesized within the body. Peptides used in therapy are often synthesized in laboratories, allowing for precise design and modification. Lab-synthesized peptides can mimic natural hormones or introduce entirely new signaling effects. This ability to custom-engineer peptides is central to their growing popularity in health optimization.

Some therapeutic peptides act like hormones, stimulating similar receptors and producing comparable effects. Others perform roles unrelated to traditional hormonal function—targeting cellular pathways involved in healing, inflammation, mitochondrial function, or even cognitive performance.

The targeted nature of peptides offers both precision and flexibility. Their structure can be modified to enhance stability, increase receptor affinity, or reduce side effects. This adaptability distinguishes peptides from natural hormones and larger proteins, which are bound by more complex structural requirements.

In short, peptides are defined by their size, signaling specificity, and customizability. They can bridge the gap between hormones and proteins—offering the precision of molecular signaling with the adaptability of modern biotechnology.

Understanding these distinctions helps clarify how peptides can be used effectively and safely. They are not interchangeable with hormones or proteins, but rather occupy a unique niche with applications in both medicine and performance enhancement. This uniqueness is what makes them such a valuable tool in the evolving world of biohacking.

Natural Production vs. Therapeutic Supplementation

Peptides are naturally synthesized in the body through tightly regulated cellular processes. Constructed from amino acids, these endogenous peptides function as signaling molecules, orchestrating a wide array of biological activities essential for maintaining homeostasis, immunity, tissue repair, metabolic balance, and hormonal regulation.

Each naturally occurring peptide plays a specific role. Some stimulate immune defenses against pathogens. Others regulate appetite, blood sugar, or stress responses. Many contribute to cell regeneration and recovery after injury. Their production is dynamic—adjusted constantly based on internal conditions and environmental inputs.

Under normal circumstances, the body's natural peptide output is sufficient for maintaining health. However, as we age or undergo physiological stress, peptide production may decline or become imbalanced. This can lead to slower recovery, reduced muscle and bone mass, impaired immune resilience, and diminished metabolic efficiency.

In these cases, therapeutic supplementation can serve as a strategic intervention. Therapeutic peptides are synthesized in controlled laboratory environments. They are either exact copies of naturally occurring peptides or modified variants engineered to enhance biological effects, increase stability, or target specific systems more precisely.

Supplementation allows for the restoration or amplification of signals that may be weakened due to age, chronic stress, or illness. For example, older individuals may benefit from peptides that support growth hormone secretion, while athletes may use peptides that enhance muscle repair or reduce inflammation post-training.

Therapeutic peptides can also be employed to address specific dysfunctions. Compounds like BPC-157 and TB-500 are used for their regenerative properties, while others like Thymosin Alpha-1 support immune modulation. By targeting precise pathways, peptide supplementation offers a level of specificity that broad interventions often lack.

However, this precision comes with responsibility. Peptides influence critical signaling systems. Improper use—whether through incorrect dosing, poor sourcing, or misaligned protocols—can lead to unintended effects. Professional oversight is strongly advised.

Another key consideration is legality and regulation. Access to therapeutic peptides varies by region. Some compounds are classified as prescription-only medications, while others are marketed for research purposes only. Compliance with local regulations is essential to ensure safe, legal access.

The distinction between natural production and supplementation lies in control. Endogenous peptides are modulated by biological feedback systems, whereas exogenous administration bypasses these controls. This makes supplementation powerful but also potentially disruptive without proper management.

Peptides are not a cure-all. They are one piece of a broader health optimization strategy that should include nutrition, exercise, sleep, and stress management. When used responsibly and strategically, they can enhance performance, support recovery, and counteract age-related decline.

Understanding this balance—between what the body already produces and what may be supplemented—is key to using peptides effectively. It is this awareness that transforms peptides from experimental compounds into targeted tools for long-term well-being.

Safety, Legality, and Regulation

Before considering peptide supplementation, it is essential to understand the critical dimensions of safety, legality, and regulation. These factors not only protect your health but also ensure that you approach peptides with responsibility and awareness.

Peptides are potent signaling agents. While they offer powerful benefits, they can also produce adverse effects if misused. Common side effects include localized reactions such as swelling or redness at the injection site. More serious outcomes, though less common, may include hormonal imbalances, unintended immune responses, or disruptions to endogenous peptide production.

Ensuring safety begins with sourcing. The peptide market is highly variable in quality. Counterfeit products, inaccurate labeling, and contaminants are significant concerns. Only purchase peptides from reputable vendors who provide verified certificates of analysis. These documents should confirm both purity and potency through third-party testing. Low-quality peptides introduce unnecessary risks and undermine any potential benefit.

Legality is another complex aspect. Peptides fall under a patchwork of regulatory classifications depending on the region. In some countries, certain peptides are tightly controlled and available only by prescription. Others may be marketed legally for research use but not for human consumption. Some peptides are permitted over the counter in select jurisdictions but remain restricted elsewhere.

Athletes face additional considerations. Many peptides are banned by organizations like the World Anti-Doping Agency (WADA) due to their potential to enhance performance. The use of these substances, even in countries where they are otherwise legal, can result in disqualification or sanctions in competitive sports.

Regulation of peptides exists in a gray area in many parts of the world. Some compounds are regulated as pharmaceuticals, while others are classified as supplements or research chemicals. This distinction affects how strictly they are controlled, labeled, and distributed. The inconsistencies make it difficult for consumers to assess product legitimacy and legality without thorough research.

Compounding this issue is the evolving nature of the regulatory landscape. As the medical and scientific communities continue to explore the clinical utility of peptides, regulatory frameworks are being updated. New rules are introduced, substances are reclassified, and previously unregulated compounds may become restricted. Keeping up with current legal standards is essential for maintaining compliance and ensuring safety.

The importance of professional guidance cannot be overstated. Healthcare providers familiar with peptide protocols can help you assess risks, select appropriate compounds, and determine correct dosing schedules. This expertise is crucial for maximizing benefit while minimizing the likelihood of complications.

Peptides hold great promise in enhancing health, recovery, and performance. But like any powerful tool, they must be used with caution. Quality control, legal compliance, and informed oversight are the foundations of safe and effective peptide use.

Understanding these principles equips you to navigate the landscape with confidence and care. Responsible use isn't optional—it's the price of entry into the world of advanced health optimization.

Why Peptides Are Biohacking Game-Changers

Peptides have emerged as one of the most transformative tools in the biohacker's toolkit—offering precise, adaptable ways to influence key biological systems and optimize human performance. Their unique ability to act as targeted messengers sets them apart from most supplements and interventions.

These short amino acid chains function as highly specific signaling agents, interacting with cellular receptors to direct responses across a wide spectrum of physiological processes. Whether regulating metabolism, enhancing immune function, supporting cognitive performance, or accelerating tissue repair, peptides operate with precision and purpose.

Unlike many natural compounds or pharmaceuticals that act broadly and often with unintended consequences, peptides can be engineered to exert focused effects. Lab-synthesized peptides can replicate natural molecules or be tailored for new biological functions—stimulating growth hormone release, boosting mitochondrial activity, promoting fat metabolism, or facilitating neuroprotection. This degree of customization allows for protocols that match individual biology and goals.

The potential for personalization is one of the defining strengths of peptides in health optimization. Every person responds differently to dietary changes, training loads, or supplements. Peptides allow biohackers to craft individualized regimens—adjusting compound selection, dosing, and timing based on personal biomarkers, goals, and feedback.

Administration methods further increase their accessibility. Peptides are available in multiple formats including subcutaneous injections, intranasal sprays, transdermal creams, and oral capsules. This range allows for flexible integration into a variety of lifestyles and comfort levels—making them viable for not only elite athletes, but also aging individuals, wellness enthusiasts, and those managing chronic conditions.

Their impact is also cumulative. When paired with foundational practices like quality nutrition, strength training, restorative sleep, and stress regulation, peptides can accelerate progress and help maintain peak performance. They are not replacements for lifestyle habits—but synergistic tools that enhance their effectiveness.

Peptides represent the future of strategic, data-driven health intervention. They offer a level of precision that aligns with the evolving ethos of biohacking: personalized, science-informed, and results-oriented.

When used responsibly, peptides empower individuals to actively shape their biology, overcome plateaus, and unlock greater resilience and vitality. Their value lies not just in what they can do, but in how intelligently they can be applied to specific, meaningful outcomes.

Their role in biohacking is only beginning to expand. As research deepens and protocols become more refined, peptides will continue to redefine what is possible in personal health optimization.

CHAPTER 2
ANTI-AGING AND LONGEVITY SUPPORT

How Peptides Influence Cellular Repair

Cellular repair is central to the body's ability to maintain health and resist the effects of aging. Every day, cells endure damage from oxidative stress, environmental toxins, metabolic byproducts, and natural biological wear. Left unchecked, this damage accumulates and contributes to age-related decline and chronic disease.

Peptides offer a powerful means of supporting and accelerating cellular repair. Acting as precision signaling molecules, peptides interact with specific cellular receptors to trigger regenerative pathways. These signals prompt cells to restore damaged structures, replace worn-out components, and maintain the integrity of their genetic and functional systems.

Certain peptides promote the repair of DNA—the molecular blueprint within each cell. DNA damage is one of the fundamental drivers of aging and cellular dysfunction. By stimulating DNA repair enzymes and enhancing genomic stability, these peptides help preserve cellular identity and reduce the risk of age-related mutations and disease.

Other peptides target mitochondrial health. Mitochondria, the energy generators of the cell, are especially vulnerable to oxidative stress and damage over time. Peptides that support mitochondrial repair can restore ATP production, improve metabolic efficiency, and slow the functional decline associated with cellular aging.

Growth factor-stimulating peptides play another critical role. These compounds encourage the release of regenerative proteins that promote cell proliferation and tissue remodeling. In damaged tissues, they accelerate the replacement of old or dysfunctional cells with newer, healthier ones—maintaining resilience across skin, muscle, nerve, and organ systems.

Peptides also aid cellular housekeeping through immune modulation. Some enhance the immune system's ability to identify and eliminate senescent or malfunctioning cells. By clearing these non-functional cells, peptides create space and biological resources for regeneration and repair.

This multi-pathway approach makes peptides uniquely effective in supporting cellular longevity. They don't merely suppress symptoms or enhance surface-level biomarkers—they interact directly with the systems that preserve cellular structure, energy, and function at a foundational level.

That said, peptides are one part of a broader strategy. Nutrition, movement, sleep, and emotional regulation remain critical to supporting natural repair mechanisms. Peptides work best when paired with habits that reduce systemic inflammation, supply essential nutrients, and create an internal environment conducive to regeneration.

Peptides help tip the balance toward restoration rather than degeneration. Through targeted activation of repair pathways, they offer the potential to slow biological aging, extend healthspan, and enhance resilience. Their ability to directly support cellular repair processes is a major reason why they are viewed as transformative tools in longevity-focused biohacking.

Combating Oxidative Stress and Mitochondrial Decline

Two of the most significant drivers of aging at the cellular level are oxidative stress and mitochondrial decline. These processes contribute to tissue degeneration, reduced energy output, and the onset of chronic disease. Peptides offer targeted solutions that support the body's ability to manage oxidative damage and preserve mitochondrial integrity—key elements in the pursuit of extended healthspan and vitality.

Oxidative stress occurs when there is an imbalance between free radicals—highly reactive molecules that damage cellular components—and the body's capacity to neutralize them with antioxidants. Persistent oxidative stress accelerates aging by impairing DNA, proteins, and cell membranes, ultimately compromising cellular performance.

Certain peptides have direct antioxidant properties, allowing them to neutralize free radicals before they cause harm. More powerfully, some peptides activate the body's own antioxidant defense systems. By upregulating the production of endogenous enzymes like superoxide dismutase, catalase, and glutathione peroxidase, these peptides enhance the body's capacity to manage oxidative load over time.

This internal signaling creates a more resilient biological environment—capable of withstanding daily oxidative challenges and reducing the accumulation of long-term cellular damage.

Mitochondrial decline is another hallmark of aging. Mitochondria generate ATP, the primary energy currency of the cell. As mitochondrial function deteriorates with age, energy production drops, metabolic efficiency decreases, and cells struggle to maintain normal function. This decline impacts everything from cognitive clarity to muscular strength and immune regulation.

Peptides support mitochondrial health on multiple fronts. Some compounds stimulate mitochondrial biogenesis, the process by which new mitochondria are formed. By increasing mitochondrial number and quality, these peptides help compensate for damaged organelles and restore energy output.

Others activate mitochondrial repair pathways—supporting the removal of dysfunctional mitochondria and enhancing the function of those that remain. This leads to more consistent ATP production and greater cellular endurance.

Peptides that reduce oxidative stress also indirectly protect mitochondria. Since mitochondria are both a source and a target of free radical damage, reducing oxidative load helps preserve mitochondrial membranes, DNA, and energy-producing machinery.

By addressing these two aging pathways simultaneously—reducing oxidative burden and revitalizing energy production—peptides provide a foundational benefit to cellular function. Their impact can be felt systemically, influencing endurance, recovery, mental clarity, skin quality, and overall vitality.

This dual action—damage reduction and energy restoration—is what makes peptides uniquely effective in longevity-focused protocols. When supported by proper nutrition, movement, sleep, and stress management, peptide strategies become a core component of biological renewal.

Understanding how to use peptides to support redox balance and mitochondrial health is essential to any serious anti-aging strategy. These are not surface-level changes, but deep interventions that support the root of biological resilience.

Skin Rejuvenation and Tissue Regeneration

Among the most visually and functionally impactful effects of peptides is their ability to support skin rejuvenation and accelerate tissue regeneration—two essential components of anti-aging strategies. These processes are not purely aesthetic; they reflect deeper systemic repair and biological resilience.

As skin ages, it naturally loses collagen—the primary protein that maintains firmness and structural integrity. The breakdown of collagen, combined with a decline in its production, results in sagging, reduced elasticity, fine lines, and wrinkles. Environmental exposure, oxidative stress, and hormonal changes further accelerate this deterioration.

Peptides offer targeted support for reversing these effects. Certain peptides stimulate fibroblasts—cells in the dermis responsible for producing collagen and elastin. By activating these pathways, peptides restore the skin's structural matrix, improving firmness and reducing visible signs of aging.

Some peptides also inhibit matrix metalloproteinases (MMPs), enzymes that degrade collagen. This dual action—stimulating production while preventing breakdown—helps rebuild skin density and slow the progression of wrinkle formation.

Hydration is another key factor in youthful skin. Hyaluronic acid, a molecule that retains water and contributes to skin plumpness, naturally diminishes with age. Specific peptides upregulate the synthesis of hyaluronic acid in the skin, improving moisture retention and giving the skin a smoother, more vibrant appearance.

The cumulative effect is not just surface-level. Peptides contribute to deeper skin health by supporting the extracellular matrix, reducing inflammation, and protecting against environmental damage. Over time, this leads to noticeable improvements in texture, tone, and resilience.

Tissue regeneration extends these benefits to a broader range of applications—muscle, joint, tendon, nerve, and even internal organ repair. Damage to tissues can arise from mechanical stress, disease, or aging. When repair processes slow down, the result is chronic pain, reduced mobility, or organ dysfunction.

Peptides involved in tissue regeneration promote the release of growth factors that drive cellular proliferation and differentiation. This speeds up the replacement of damaged or senescent cells with new, functional tissue. Peptides like BPC-157 and TB-500 are well-documented for their roles in accelerating recovery from injuries, enhancing connective tissue integrity, and supporting systemic healing.

In parallel, peptides can regulate the immune environment during healing. Excessive inflammation can hinder tissue repair, delay recovery, or even cause additional damage. By modulating inflammatory pathways and promoting immune resolution, certain peptides ensure that the regenerative process proceeds efficiently and without unnecessary interference.

Used consistently and as part of a well-rounded protocol, peptides can significantly enhance both surface-level aesthetics and deep tissue health. They are not isolated beauty agents but foundational tools for restoring function and supporting long-term regeneration.

Whether the goal is to improve skin elasticity or to accelerate healing after injury, peptides offer a versatile and effective solution rooted in biology. Their ability to target both cosmetic and structural concerns makes them an indispensable part of any anti-aging and longevity approach.

Promoting Youthful Energy and Vitality

Sustaining energy and vitality as we age is a core focus of anti-aging strategies—and peptides offer a powerful means to support this goal at a cellular and systemic level. Vitality is not simply about feeling awake or energized in the moment. It reflects the underlying efficiency of cellular processes, the stability of hormonal systems, and the body's ability to repair and regenerate.

As we grow older, cellular efficiency often declines. Mitochondria—the organelles responsible for producing ATP, the energy currency of the cell—become damaged or dysfunctional. This mitochondrial decline leads to reduced energy production, physical fatigue, slower recovery, and a general sense of diminished vitality.

Peptides offer a targeted solution. Some compounds stimulate mitochondrial biogenesis, increasing the number of energy-producing organelles within cells. More mitochondria means more capacity to generate ATP, resulting in higher baseline energy levels and improved endurance.

Other peptides support mitochondrial repair, restoring the function of existing mitochondria and improving energy output across multiple tissues. By repairing oxidative damage and boosting metabolic efficiency, these peptides help restore a more youthful baseline of energy and resilience.

In parallel, peptides contribute to hormonal optimization, another key component of sustained vitality. Hormones regulate metabolism, mood, motivation, and physical performance. As we age, natural hormone production—such as testosterone, estrogen, DHEA, and growth hormone—often declines, resulting in fatigue, mood instability, and decreased physical capacity.

Certain peptides can stimulate the body's own hormone production. For example, growth hormone secretagogues encourage the pituitary gland to release growth hormone, supporting muscle retention, fat metabolism, and overall vigor. Others influence the hypothalamic-pituitary-gonadal axis, indirectly supporting balanced testosterone and estrogen levels.

These hormonal adjustments support not only physical energy, but also mental clarity, motivation, and emotional stability—hallmarks of what we commonly associate with youthful vitality.

Recovery also plays a critical role. As recovery slows with age, minor stressors—like physical exertion or injury—can drain energy reserves and delay return to baseline. Peptides that support tissue repair and inflammation modulation help shorten recovery time, reduce soreness, and maintain functional capacity across daily activities.

This triad—mitochondrial function, hormonal balance, and recovery speed—underlies sustainable vitality. Peptides that enhance these systems provide meaningful, measurable support for maintaining performance, reducing fatigue, and extending the healthspan of body and mind.

However, peptides should always be integrated into a comprehensive lifestyle plan. Nutrition, movement, rest, and stress regulation remain foundational. Peptides serve to accelerate progress, not replace core habits.

Used wisely, peptides allow for a restoration of energy levels typically associated with youth—without relying on stimulants or unsustainable hacks. They act at the biological roots of fatigue and performance decline, making them one of the most effective tools for preserving vitality over time.

Popular Anti-Aging Peptides to Know

As interest in longevity and performance optimization grows, certain peptides have gained recognition for their ability to counteract age-related decline and support regenerative processes. These compounds are widely used in the biohacking community for their cellular-level effects on vitality, appearance, and resilience. Understanding the function and application of these peptides can help you make informed choices within a structured health optimization strategy.

Epitalon is one of the most studied peptides in the context of lifespan extension. It is known to stimulate the activity of telomerase, an enzyme that maintains the length of telomeres—protective caps on the ends of chromosomes that shorten with each cell division. Telomere shortening is associated with biological aging and cellular dysfunction. By supporting telomere preservation, Epitalon may slow down cellular aging and contribute to extended healthspan.

GHK-Cu, a copper peptide naturally found in human plasma, has strong regenerative and cosmetic benefits. It promotes collagen and elastin synthesis, making it a standout for skin repair and anti-aging applications. Additionally, GHK-Cu has antioxidant and anti-inflammatory effects and may assist in wound healing and tissue remodeling. Its role in restoring skin tone, reducing wrinkles, and improving overall skin quality has made it a staple in both peptide therapy and high-end skincare formulations.

Thymosin Beta-4 (TB-500) supports tissue repair and regeneration, particularly in muscle, connective tissue, and blood vessels. It enhances angiogenesis, the formation of new blood vessels, and modulates the immune response to reduce excessive inflammation. TB-500 is often used to accelerate recovery from physical injuries, surgeries, or intense training, making it valuable for maintaining mobility and resilience as the body ages.

CJC-1295 is a growth hormone-releasing hormone (GHRH) analog that stimulates the pituitary gland to increase growth hormone secretion. Rather than supplying exogenous hormones, it encourages the body's own production through natural pathways. This can lead to improved energy levels, fat metabolism, sleep quality, and muscle retention—all of which tend to decline with age. When paired with Ipamorelin, a growth hormone secretagogue, its effects can be amplified without significant spikes in cortisol or prolactin.

Each of these peptides addresses a different dimension of aging—from genomic stability and skin regeneration to hormone regulation and recovery enhancement. The right peptide choice depends on individual goals, health status, and response to therapy.

It's important to view peptides as part of a broader health optimization plan. They are not replacements for foundational practices like nutrient-dense eating, physical activity, restorative sleep, and stress reduction. Instead, peptides should be used to support and enhance these pillars—amplifying your body's ability to repair, regenerate, and perform at its best.

Professional oversight is also essential. Dosing, sourcing, and protocol design should be guided by a qualified provider who understands both the biological mechanisms and your personal health profile.

As we move forward, we'll continue exploring these and other anti-aging peptides—diving into their mechanisms, use cases, and how to incorporate them safely into a personalized longevity strategy.

CHAPTER 3

FAT LOSS AND METABOLIC ENHANCEMENT

Metabolic Peptides and Their Role in Weight Regulation

Metabolic peptides represent a powerful class of compounds capable of influencing several key processes involved in weight regulation. These peptides modulate energy production, fat metabolism, and appetite control—factors that together determine body composition and metabolic health.

At the core of metabolic regulation is energy expenditure, driven primarily by mitochondrial activity. Certain peptides stimulate mitochondrial biogenesis, increasing both the number and efficiency of mitochondria within cells. This leads to elevated basal metabolic rate (BMR), which in turn boosts calorie burn—even at rest. Enhanced energy production supports both fat loss and increased endurance, providing a metabolic environment conducive to body recomposition.

Beyond energy production, peptides can also target fat mobilization. Some compounds directly promote lipolysis, the breakdown of stored triglycerides into free fatty acids. By enhancing this process, these peptides facilitate the release of fat from adipose tissue, making it available for use as energy. Over time, this contributes to reductions in body fat percentage and improved metabolic flexibility.

Equally important is appetite regulation. Metabolic peptides can influence hunger and satiety signals by interacting with receptors in the hypothalamus—the brain's control center for energy balance. Certain peptides promote the sensation of fullness and reduce food cravings, supporting lower caloric intake without the psychological burden of restrictive dieting. This neuromodulatory effect makes it easier to maintain a caloric deficit necessary for fat loss.

Together, these mechanisms form a multi-faceted approach to weight regulation. Increased energy output, enhanced fat breakdown, and reduced caloric intake work in concert to promote sustainable fat loss while preserving lean mass.

However, these benefits must be understood in context. Metabolic peptides are not a substitute for lifestyle changes. Without proper nutrition, exercise, sleep, and stress management, their effects are limited. Used strategically, peptides can amplify progress, improve metabolic efficiency, and provide a powerful edge—but only when combined with foundational health practices.

Additionally, not all metabolic peptides are appropriate for all individuals. Health status, existing metabolic conditions, and individual response variability must be taken into account. Protocols should be customized and monitored by a qualified healthcare provider to ensure safety and optimize results.

Peptides offer an advanced, biologically aligned way to support fat loss and metabolic health. By enhancing mitochondrial function, stimulating lipolysis, and regulating appetite, they unlock new possibilities for individuals seeking more efficient and sustainable weight management.

As we move deeper into this chapter, we'll explore specific peptides used in metabolic enhancement, how to integrate them into a targeted plan, and what to expect in terms of results and safety.

Targeting Stubborn Fat Through Hormonal Pathways

Stubborn fat is often resistant to traditional weight loss efforts—persisting even with disciplined nutrition and consistent training. This resistance is largely influenced by hormonal signals that regulate fat storage and mobilization. Peptides, through their ability to interact with key hormonal pathways, offer a targeted strategy for addressing this challenge.

Hormones act as the body's command signals, directing where and how energy is stored or released. Certain hormones—most notably insulin, cortisol, and estrogen—can drive fat accumulation in specific regions, making it difficult to eliminate fat from areas like the abdomen, hips, or thighs without addressing the underlying hormonal influences.

Insulin is central to metabolic balance and fat storage. When insulin levels are elevated, the body shifts into a fat-storing mode, particularly in visceral regions. Some peptides improve insulin sensitivity, allowing cells to respond to lower levels of insulin while maintaining stable blood glucose. As insulin levels normalize, the metabolic environment becomes less prone to fat storage and more favorable to fat breakdown, especially in areas typically resistant to change.

Cortisol, commonly referred to as the "stress hormone," is another major factor. Chronic stress elevates cortisol, which can increase abdominal fat storage and inhibit fat breakdown. Peptides that support cortisol regulation help reduce this stress-induced fat accumulation. By modulating the body's stress response and stabilizing cortisol rhythms, these peptides contribute to a more balanced metabolic profile.

Estrogen, especially in women, plays a role in region-specific fat storage. Higher estrogen levels are associated with fat accumulation in the hips, thighs, and buttocks. Peptides that promote hormonal balance—rather than artificially suppressing hormone levels—can help redistribute fat storage patterns and reduce accumulation in estrogen-sensitive areas.

Beyond hormonal modulation, certain peptides actively promote lipolysis, the breakdown of stored triglycerides into usable energy. This process not only helps reduce overall fat stores, but also enables the body to mobilize fat from hard-to-target areas. By stimulating lipolytic activity in adipose tissue, these peptides support the body's capacity to utilize stubborn fat as fuel.

This hormonal and cellular synergy makes peptides a highly effective complement to a weight loss program. They work at the root level—restoring hormonal balance and improving metabolic signaling—rather than simply masking symptoms or forcing short-term results.

However, even with their powerful effects, peptides must be integrated into a comprehensive lifestyle framework. Fat loss depends on multiple factors: caloric intake, energy output, sleep quality, nutrient status, and mental well-being. Peptides enhance and accelerate progress but do not replace foundational habits.

Protocols must be individualized, based on metabolic needs, hormonal profile, and health history. Oversight from a qualified healthcare provider ensures both effectiveness and safety—especially when using peptides that influence complex endocrine systems.

Stubborn fat does not respond well to generic solutions. Peptides offer a strategic, biology-aligned approach—making it possible to finally shift resistant fat stores by correcting the hormonal signals that keep them in place.

Appetite Suppression and Satiety Signals

Managing hunger and achieving sustained satiety are central to effective weight regulation. While willpower alone often fails over the long term, peptides offer a biologically intelligent approach to appetite control—targeting the internal signaling systems that regulate when and how much we eat.

Appetite is orchestrated by a delicate balance of hormonal messengers that communicate between the gut, the brain, and peripheral tissues. Signals of hunger and fullness are continuously adjusted based on nutrient status, energy needs, circadian rhythms, and stress. Disruptions in these signals—whether from chronic dieting, inflammation, or metabolic imbalances—can drive overeating and weight gain.

Peptides can help recalibrate this system. One major target is ghrelin, often called the "hunger hormone." Ghrelin is secreted primarily by the stomach and activates receptors in the hypothalamus to stimulate appetite. Certain peptides can antagonize ghrelin signaling, binding to its receptors without activating them. This prevents ghrelin from triggering hunger, helping to blunt excessive food cravings and reduce overall calorie intake.

Other peptides work by enhancing satiety hormones, such as peptide YY (PYY) and glucagon-like peptide-1 (GLP-1). These hormones are released by the gut after food intake and send strong signals to the brain indicating fullness. Peptides that stimulate the release of PYY or mimic GLP-1 activity increase the sensation of fullness after meals, making it easier to eat less without discomfort.

Another effective strategy is to slow gastric emptying—the rate at which food exits the stomach. Certain peptides can delay this process, prolonging the physical sensation of fullness and reducing the urge to eat soon after a meal. This physiological delay can be particularly useful for curbing snacking and supporting portion control.

Together, these mechanisms create a sustained and natural reduction in appetite. Unlike stimulant-based appetite suppressants, peptides modulate internal signals in alignment with the body's biological rhythms, making them better suited for long-term use and metabolic support.

However, appetite suppression is not inherently a solution. Hunger is a critical feedback mechanism, and ignoring or excessively suppressing it can lead to nutritional deficiencies, hormonal disruption, and emotional dysregulation. The goal is not to eliminate hunger altogether, but to normalize appetite cues—supporting a balanced relationship with food.

Peptides that regulate appetite work best when paired with nutrient-dense meals, proper hydration, physical activity, and adequate sleep. When these fundamentals are in place, peptides can amplify satiety signals and make adherence to a healthful eating plan more sustainable.

Protocols should always be personalized and professionally guided, especially for individuals with a history of disordered eating or metabolic conditions.

When used responsibly, peptides provide powerful support for regulating appetite and enhancing satiety—two often-overlooked keys to long-term fat loss success. They allow individuals to work with their biology, not against it, creating the internal environment necessary for sustainable, healthy weight management.

Improving Insulin Sensitivity and Glucose Balance

Insulin sensitivity and glucose regulation are foundational to metabolic health and play a central role in body composition, energy utilization, and fat storage. When these processes are disrupted, the body becomes prone to weight gain, inflammation, and metabolic disorders. Peptides offer a strategic means to support insulin function and maintain stable glucose dynamics—making them valuable tools in fat loss and metabolic enhancement.

Insulin is the hormone responsible for facilitating the uptake of glucose into cells, where it can be used for energy or stored for later use. After carbohydrate intake, glucose enters the bloodstream, prompting insulin release from the pancreas. In a healthy system, insulin effectively delivers glucose to muscle, fat, and liver cells, keeping blood sugar levels in check.

Insulin sensitivity describes how responsive cells are to this process. In insulin-sensitive individuals, cells readily absorb glucose when insulin is present. In contrast, insulin resistance occurs when cells fail to respond efficiently, causing glucose and insulin levels to remain elevated. Over time, this state can lead to chronic hyperinsulinemia, fat accumulation—particularly visceral fat—and conditions like metabolic syndrome or type 2 diabetes.

Peptides can improve insulin sensitivity through multiple mechanisms. Some peptides enhance insulin receptor signaling, increasing cellular responsiveness to insulin. This allows glucose to be cleared from the bloodstream more efficiently and reduces the need for excess insulin release.

Other peptides work by reducing systemic inflammation, which plays a key role in the development of insulin resistance. By dampening inflammatory cytokines and supporting immune regulation, these peptides help restore metabolic balance at the cellular level.

In addition to improving insulin function, certain peptides also aid in stabilizing glucose levels. Some peptides delay carbohydrate absorption in the digestive tract, slowing the entry of glucose into the bloodstream and preventing post-meal blood sugar spikes. This helps minimize insulin demand and reduces the risk of metabolic overload.

Other peptides promote regulated insulin secretion—stimulating insulin release in a glucose-dependent manner. This means insulin is released when needed, but not excessively, supporting balanced blood sugar without contributing to fat storage or insulin resistance.

These effects create a more stable internal environment—marked by improved energy regulation, reduced fat storage, and decreased cravings linked to blood sugar fluctuations.

Still, peptides must be integrated into a comprehensive metabolic plan. Their effectiveness depends heavily on foundational practices like nutrient-dense eating, consistent movement, high-quality sleep, and stress control. Peptides support and amplify these efforts—they do not replace them.

Insulin and glucose are essential physiological systems that must be modulated, not suppressed. The goal is not to eliminate these signals but to restore their natural efficiency. Peptides offer precision and personalization in this effort, helping correct dysfunction while maintaining biological balance.

Used wisely, peptides can enhance metabolic resilience, support fat loss, and prevent the cascade of health issues associated with impaired glucose handling. When tailored to individual needs and guided by professional oversight, they are among the most impactful tools for improving metabolic health at its core.

Peptide Stacks for Body Recomposition

Body recomposition—the process of simultaneously reducing fat mass and increasing lean muscle—is a goal that demands a strategic blend of training, nutrition, recovery, and hormonal optimization. Peptides offer a precise and synergistic approach to accelerate this transformation. When thoughtfully combined, or "stacked," peptides can target multiple physiological mechanisms at once to support enhanced metabolic function and muscle development.

A peptide stack is a curated combination of peptides, each selected to influence a different yet complementary process. In the context of body recomposition, the primary objectives are to boost muscle protein synthesis, promote fat oxidation, optimize hormonal balance, and improve nutrient partitioning—how the body directs calories toward muscle growth rather than fat storage.

A foundational stack for recomposition often starts with CJC-1295 paired with Ipamorelin. CJC-1295 is a growth hormone-releasing hormone (GHRH) analog, while Ipamorelin is a growth hormone secretagogue. Together, they enhance natural growth hormone pulsatility without significantly affecting cortisol or prolactin. This dynamic duo increases IGF-1 production, supporting muscle repair, fat metabolism, and recovery.

To further shift the metabolic scale toward fat loss, AOD-9604 is commonly added. AOD-9604 is a modified fragment of human growth hormone designed specifically to stimulate lipolysis and inhibit lipogenesis—effectively promoting fat breakdown while minimizing fat formation. Unlike full hGH, it lacks significant anabolic activity, making it ideal for fat-targeted effects without muscle water retention or joint stiffness.

Another high-impact addition is IGF-1 LR3, a long-acting analog of insulin-like growth factor-1. IGF-1 LR3 plays a pivotal role in muscle cell proliferation and glucose uptake, helping direct nutrients into muscle tissue rather than fat stores. It also improves insulin sensitivity, which can aid in regulating energy metabolism and enhancing the anabolic environment post-training.

Depending on individual needs, additional peptides may be integrated to fine-tune the stack. Peptides that modulate appetite, enhance mitochondrial function, or reduce inflammation can offer supportive benefits during periods of caloric restriction or intense training.

It's important to emphasize that peptide stacks are not plug-and-play solutions. Each person's physiology, training intensity, and dietary structure will influence how they respond. Stacks should be tailored, cycled, and closely monitored—preferably with support from a practitioner experienced in peptide therapy.

Moreover, no stack will be effective in the absence of fundamentals. Adequate protein intake, resistance training, sleep quality, and stress control remain essential pillars of body recomposition. Peptides act as accelerators—not replacements—for these foundations.

When used with precision and responsibility, peptide stacks offer a powerful tool for reshaping body composition. By combining pathways that target fat loss, muscle growth, and metabolic efficiency, these stacks can deliver results that go beyond what is achievable through training and diet alone.

As we continue exploring the peptide landscape, we'll further unpack how to build effective protocols, adjust them to changing goals, and use them safely as part of a long-term strategy for body transformation and metabolic resilience.

CHAPTER 4
MUSCLE GROWTH AND PHYSICAL RECOVERY

How Peptides Aid Muscle Repair and Growth

Muscle growth and repair are driven by a cascade of biological processes activated in response to stress, especially resistance training. When muscle fibers experience micro-damage from exercise, the body initiates a recovery process that not only repairs the tissue but often results in adaptation—growth, strength gains, and enhanced resilience. Peptides play a key role in optimizing this response by influencing growth signaling, hormone release, protein synthesis, and tissue regeneration.

One of the primary classes of peptides involved in muscle development is growth hormone-releasing peptides (GHRPs). These peptides stimulate the pituitary gland to release growth hormone (GH)—a key anabolic hormone that supports muscle protein synthesis, cell repair, and fat metabolism. Increased GH levels promote tissue regeneration, enhance amino acid uptake in muscles, and accelerate recovery.

CJC-1295, a growth hormone-releasing hormone (GHRH) analog, is known for its ability to sustain elevated GH and insulin-like growth factor 1 (IGF-1) levels without overstimulating the endocrine system. CJC-1295 improves recovery between workouts, increases lean muscle mass, and supports fat loss—making it ideal for body recomposition and performance enhancement.

Ipamorelin, a selective GHRP, also triggers GH release but without the cortisol or prolactin elevation commonly seen with older peptides. It allows for GH stimulation with a cleaner side effect profile, making it a well-tolerated option for those focused on recovery and hypertrophy.

Beyond hormonal modulation, peptides support angiogenesis, the formation of new capillaries in muscle tissue. Increased capillary density improves oxygen and nutrient delivery to muscles during training and recovery, accelerating the repair of microtears and supporting mitochondrial function. Peptides that stimulate angiogenesis help create a more efficient environment for muscle regeneration.

Another peptide of interest is follistatin, which works by inhibiting myostatin—a protein that limits muscle growth. By suppressing myostatin, follistatin removes a natural barrier to hypertrophy, enabling greater muscle protein synthesis and enhanced muscle volume over time. This mechanism is particularly attractive to athletes and aging individuals seeking to preserve or build lean mass.

Peptides also support recovery through anti-inflammatory and cellular repair pathways. By reducing muscle inflammation and oxidative stress, peptides help shorten the downtime between training sessions, allowing for more frequent and intense workouts without overtraining.

Despite their powerful effects, peptides are not a substitute for core practices. Training intensity, nutrient timing, protein intake, and sleep quality remain the foundation of any effective muscle-building plan. Peptides serve to amplify these efforts, not replace them.

Proper use involves personalization—aligning the peptide type, dosage, and cycle length with specific training goals and physiological needs. All protocols should be guided by a knowledgeable provider to avoid misuse and maximize results.

When integrated intelligently, peptides offer a significant edge in both muscle growth and physical recovery. They enable the body to repair faster, grow stronger, and adapt more efficiently—supporting sustainable gains and long-term performance. As we continue our exploration, we'll examine additional peptides that enhance muscular development and recovery in even more targeted ways.

Supporting Collagen Synthesis and Tendon Strength

While much attention is given to muscle hypertrophy and fat loss, collagen synthesis and tendon integrity are equally critical components of sustainable physical performance. Tendons serve as the essential links between muscle and bone—transmitting force, maintaining structural alignment, and withstanding the high mechanical demands of movement. Peptides that enhance collagen production and support tendon strength can dramatically reduce injury risk and improve long-term functional capacity.

Collagen is the most abundant structural protein in the body. It provides tensile strength and flexibility to skin, joints, bones, and connective tissues—especially tendons and ligaments. Over time, or under repetitive stress, collagen can degrade. Aging, inflammation, overtraining, and poor nutrition can all compromise collagen integrity, making tendons more prone to strain, microtears, or rupture.

Peptides such as BPC-157 have shown strong potential in enhancing collagen synthesis and tissue repair. BPC-157 promotes the proliferation of fibroblasts—the cells responsible for producing collagen—and accelerates wound healing in tendons, muscles, and ligaments. It supports the remodeling of injured tissue while reinforcing its strength, making it particularly valuable in the recovery of tendinopathies or chronic overuse injuries.

Another powerful peptide, GHK-Cu, also contributes to collagen regeneration. Originally noted for its skin-repair properties, GHK-Cu stimulates collagen production at the cellular level and improves tissue elasticity and tensile strength. Although most commonly used in dermatology, its regenerative effects may extend to deeper connective tissues, supporting structural integrity beyond the skin.

TB-500, a synthetic version of thymosin beta-4, plays a complementary role by promoting angiogenesis, or the growth of new blood vessels. Tendons typically have poor vascularity, limiting their capacity to receive oxygen and nutrients. By enhancing blood flow, TB-500 improves the metabolic environment around tendon tissue—supporting both healing and resilience.

Together, these peptides help create a pro-repair environment in soft tissues, enabling faster recovery from mechanical strain and promoting the long-term durability of connective structures. For athletes, lifters, and active individuals, this translates to better training continuity, reduced downtime, and lower risk of chronic injury.

However, peptides should be integrated into a holistic recovery and performance plan. Adequate intake of amino acids, vitamin C, and collagen-specific nutrients (like glycine and proline) is essential to supply the raw materials needed for collagen synthesis. Resistance training with progressive loading also helps stimulate the mechanical signaling required for tendon adaptation.

It's important to recognize that tendon remodeling occurs more slowly than muscle growth. Patience, consistency, and smart load management are key. Peptides can accelerate the healing timeline and strengthen tissue under repair, but they cannot bypass the natural pace of biological adaptation.

Used strategically, peptides like BPC-157, GHK-Cu, and TB-500 offer a powerful way to reinforce tendon health and optimize the structural foundation of physical performance. By addressing tissue resilience at its root, they help safeguard longevity in training and athletic endeavors—enhancing recovery, durability, and functional strength over time.

Workout Recovery, Injury Healing, and Performance Boosting

I Effective training isn't just about what happens in the gym—it's about how the body recovers, adapts, and performs under repeated physical demands. Peptides offer targeted support for each phase of this cycle, enhancing recovery speed, improving injury resilience, and elevating performance capacity. When integrated thoughtfully, they provide a strategic advantage for athletes, fitness enthusiasts, and anyone pursuing long-term physical excellence.

Workout recovery is the foundation of muscular development. During intense physical activity, muscle fibers experience micro-damage that must be repaired for adaptation to occur. Growth hormone plays a central role in this process, stimulating tissue regeneration, protein synthesis, and cellular recovery.

Peptides like CJC-1295 and Ipamorelin boost endogenous growth hormone release without overstimulating other hormonal pathways. Together, they enhance anabolic signaling post-exercise, accelerating muscle recovery, improving sleep quality, and reducing post-workout fatigue. This enables more frequent training with reduced risk of overtraining.

Injury healing is another domain where peptides shine. Soft tissue injuries, whether acute (like sprains or muscle tears) or chronic (such as tendonitis or ligament strain), often stall progress and undermine consistency. Peptides such as BPC-157 and TB-500 are known for their regenerative and anti-inflammatory properties.

BPC-157 supports tendon and ligament healing by increasing blood flow, promoting collagen production, and enhancing fibroblast activity. It is particularly effective in treating overuse injuries and accelerating post-operative recovery. TB-500, through its role in angiogenesis and cell migration, supports rapid repair of muscle, fascia, and joint tissues—making it ideal for widespread or systemic soft tissue recovery.

Beyond repair, peptides can also elevate physical performance. One way is through improving oxygen delivery via increased red blood cell production. Certain peptides indirectly enhance the body's erythropoietin (EPO) response, supporting aerobic endurance and delaying fatigue in high-intensity efforts.

Additionally, peptides that modulate IGF-1 levels (a critical downstream hormone of growth hormone) support muscle hypertrophy, neuromuscular efficiency, and power output. This is especially beneficial in strength and hypertrophy training protocols.

However, peptides do not replace the fundamentals of periodized training, nutrient timing, hydration, and sleep. They are accelerators of adaptation—tools to enhance recovery windows, support tissue integrity, and optimize natural hormone rhythms.

Individual variability must also be respected. Peptides interact with your unique biology, training intensity, and lifestyle inputs. Responses may vary, and protocols should be adjusted accordingly with regular progress assessments and professional supervision.

Used intelligently, peptides offer a biological edge that supports faster recovery, resilient tissue health, and sustained performance gains. They allow the body to not only train harder—but also recover smarter and perform stronger. As we explore further, we'll continue examining how peptides can be aligned with your goals for strength, endurance, and total body optimization.

Balancing Growth with Inflammation Control

Effective muscle growth and recovery hinge not only on anabolic stimulation but also on the strategic regulation of inflammation. Inflammation is essential for tissue repair, yet when uncontrolled, it can impair recovery, promote catabolism, and increase the risk of injury. Peptides offer a powerful tool for maintaining this delicate balance—supporting growth while modulating inflammation to ensure optimal recovery and performance.

Acute inflammation is the body's immediate response to physical stress or injury. Following intense exercise, microtears in muscle fibers trigger localized inflammation, marked by increased blood flow, immune cell activity, and nutrient delivery. This controlled response facilitates repair, adaptation, and muscle hypertrophy.

However, when inflammation becomes chronic or excessive, it shifts from being regenerative to degenerative. Prolonged inflammatory signaling can delay healing, disrupt anabolic signaling, degrade connective tissue, and promote fatigue or overtraining syndromes.

Peptides such as BPC-157 and TB-500 help maintain this balance by modulating inflammatory cytokines—increasing anti-inflammatory markers like IL-10 while suppressing pro-inflammatory signals such as TNF-α and IL-6. This targeted regulation allows for continued immune support and tissue repair without tipping into chronic inflammation.

BPC-157 supports angiogenesis, tissue remodeling, and fibroblast activity while simultaneously dampening inflammatory pathways. It reduces oxidative stress in damaged areas and promotes the regeneration of tendons, muscles, and ligaments—making it especially useful for athletes prone to soft tissue strain.

TB-500 enhances cell migration and blood vessel formation, improving the delivery of oxygen and nutrients to recovering tissues. It modulates immune activity to prevent inflammatory overload while supporting cellular regeneration. These actions create an ideal internal environment for both growth and restoration.

Importantly, these peptides also influence the production of growth factors like VEGF, IGF-1, and FGF. These proteins are crucial for satellite cell activation, myogenesis, and the structural adaptation of muscle tissue—linking inflammation resolution with muscle repair.

But peptides are not a substitute for foundational recovery strategies. Overtraining, nutrient deficiencies, and insufficient rest can overwhelm even the most effective peptide protocols. Adequate protein intake, sleep, hydration, and training periodization are essential to support natural inflammatory cycles and optimize tissue regeneration.

Furthermore, it's crucial to understand that inflammation is not the enemy—it is a biological signal that initiates repair. Suppressing it entirely can impair adaptation. The goal is not to eliminate inflammation, but to manage it with precision, allowing the body to recover faster without compromising long-term performance or resilience.

When used responsibly, peptides such as BPC-157 and TB-500 provide a unique ability to support muscle growth while preventing inflammatory overload. They enhance recovery quality, reduce downtime, and help maintain the structural integrity of muscle and connective tissue—making them a powerful ally in any performance-driven regimen.

As we continue exploring the utility of peptides in fitness and recovery, this balance between anabolism and inflammation control remains a cornerstone for building strength, durability, and long-term physical health.

Popular Peptides in the Fitness World

In the evolving landscape of performance enhancement, peptides have emerged as some of the most sought-after tools for those pursuing gains in muscle growth, recovery, fat loss, and physical resilience. Widely used by bodybuilders, athletes, and biohackers alike, these compounds offer targeted benefits through biological pathways that align closely with fitness goals. Understanding the most popular peptides and how they function can help guide informed, responsible use.

CJC-1295 is a growth hormone-releasing hormone (GHRH) analog that stimulates the pituitary gland to release growth hormone in pulses—closely mimicking the body's natural rhythm. By increasing growth hormone and IGF-1 levels, CJC-1295 supports muscle hypertrophy, fat metabolism, and recovery enhancement. It's often stacked with Ipamorelin, a selective growth hormone secretagogue that delivers similar benefits without elevating cortisol or prolactin. Together, they form a synergistic pair that boosts anabolism and tissue regeneration without overloading the endocrine system.

BPC-157 is known for its potent regenerative properties. It promotes tendon, ligament, and muscle repair, supports blood vessel formation, and reduces inflammation at injury sites. BPC-157 is widely used by strength athletes and those with chronic soft tissue issues, as it helps reduce downtime and accelerates healing from both overuse and acute injuries.

TB-500, a synthetic version of thymosin beta-4, complements BPC-157 by improving cell migration and flexibility through its effects on actin regulation and extracellular matrix repair. It supports injury recovery at a systemic level and may enhance joint mobility and muscular pliability, particularly valuable for dynamic athletes or those in mobility-demanding disciplines.

AOD-9604 is a modified fragment of human growth hormone designed specifically to stimulate lipolysis while inhibiting lipogenesis. Its fat-targeting mechanism makes it a popular option for athletes and fitness enthusiasts looking to shed fat while preserving muscle mass—without the anabolic effects or water retention associated with full hGH.

MK-677 (Ibutamoren) is a non-peptide secretagogue that mimics ghrelin and stimulates growth hormone release. Uniquely, it's orally bioavailable, offering convenience for users averse to injections. MK-677 is favored for its ability to support lean mass gain, improved sleep quality, and enhanced recovery, making it especially popular during bulking phases or recomposition cycles.

Each of these compounds targets a specific physiological mechanism—from hormonal stimulation to tissue healing to fat metabolism. When used strategically, they can accelerate fitness progress beyond what is achievable with training and nutrition alone.

That said, peptides are not substitutes for foundational practices. Proper training, nutrient timing, sleep hygiene, hydration, and recovery protocols remain the pillars of athletic progress. Peptides serve as adjuncts, helping to fine-tune recovery and growth processes already set in motion by smart lifestyle choices.

It's also vital to acknowledge that many peptides are still in early or experimental stages of research. Long-term safety profiles and optimal dosing strategies are not fully established, and sourcing must be handled with extreme caution. Usage should be overseen by a knowledgeable provider familiar with peptide therapy, with individual responses monitored regularly.

When integrated responsibly, peptides like CJC-1295, Ipamorelin, BPC-157, TB-500, AOD-9604, and MK-677 provide significant leverage in the pursuit of strength, recovery, body composition, and overall athletic longevity. As we move forward, we'll continue unpacking how these compounds can be aligned with precise training goals, phased cycles, and long-term performance plans.

CHAPTER 5

SLEEP OPTIMIZATION AND CIRCADIAN HEALTH

The Link Between Sleep Quality and Peptide Production

Sleep is a foundational pillar of health—essential for recovery, hormonal regulation, metabolic balance, and cognitive function. Among its many physiological benefits, sleep also plays a vital role in the synthesis, release, and regulation of key peptides. Conversely, peptides themselves influence sleep architecture and circadian timing, creating a bidirectional relationship that directly impacts performance, recovery, and longevity.

One of the most significant connections between sleep and peptide production involves growth hormone (GH). The majority of natural GH secretion occurs during slow-wave sleep (SWS)—the deepest and most restorative phase of the sleep cycle. Peptides that stimulate GH release, such as CJC-1295 and Ipamorelin, are most effective when aligned with this sleep phase. If sleep quality is compromised—due to stress, circadian misalignment, or stimulants—GH secretion may be blunted, weakening the body's repair and recovery capacity.

Another peptide with a circadian influence is ghrelin, which helps regulate appetite and metabolism. Ghrelin levels typically rise at night and fall during the day. Poor sleep or irregular sleep patterns can disrupt ghrelin rhythms, increasing hunger cues and contributing to poor metabolic control, late-night cravings, and body fat accumulation.

On the wakefulness side of the equation, orexin (hypocretin) is a neuropeptide that governs alertness and sleep-wake transitions. Imbalances in orexin signaling are strongly associated with narcolepsy and disrupted sleep regulation. Emerging peptide therapies that modulate orexin pathways are being studied for their potential to enhance sleep stability and manage circadian disorders.

While not a peptide, melatonin—the master hormone of the sleep-wake cycle—is heavily influenced by peptide-driven processes. Some peptides may help support melatonin synthesis indirectly by stabilizing the internal biological clock or reducing inflammation that disrupts hormonal rhythms.

This interplay shows that sleep is both a regulator and a beneficiary of peptide activity. Without adequate sleep, peptide-dependent repair and anabolic processes are impaired. Without sufficient peptide activity—particularly GH and neuropeptide signaling—sleep quality, depth, and consistency suffer.

But peptide balance doesn't exist in isolation. Sleep quality is shaped by a wide range of lifestyle and environmental inputs—light exposure, caffeine intake, blue light from screens, eating patterns, alcohol, psychological stress, and circadian misalignment all interfere with deep, peptide-supportive sleep.

Optimizing sleep means targeting all of these variables while potentially incorporating peptide support when appropriate. For example, aligning GH-releasing peptide protocols with bedtime may improve outcomes, while using peptides that regulate inflammation and stress response (like BPC-157) may also enhance sleep quality indirectly.

The key is synergy: peptides and sleep must work in tandem to support total recovery and optimal physiology. Neglecting sleep undermines peptide efficacy. Enhancing sleep while leveraging peptide signaling, however, creates a powerful feedback loop of growth, balance, and regeneration.

As we continue our exploration of sleep optimization and circadian health, we'll delve into targeted strategies and specific peptides that can enhance sleep quality, support hormonal rhythm, and promote deeper, more restorative rest.

Peptides That Support Deep, Restful Sleep

Quality sleep is not just about duration—it's about depth and consistency. The deepest stages of non-REM sleep, especially delta-wave sleep, are when the body engages in its most intensive repair, immune regulation, and hormonal recalibration. Certain peptides offer targeted support for enhancing sleep architecture, improving the quality—not just the quantity—of rest. These compounds help synchronize circadian rhythms, support hormone release, and promote neurological calm, making them valuable tools for optimizing recovery and overall well-being.

One of the most notable peptides for sleep is DSIP (Delta Sleep-Inducing Peptide). Discovered for its ability to enhance slow-wave (delta) sleep, DSIP helps regulate sleep cycles by modulating stress-related neurochemicals such as corticotropin and norepinephrine. Its influence on the hypothalamic-pituitary-adrenal (HPA) axis may reduce nighttime arousal, making it particularly beneficial for individuals struggling with insomnia or fragmented sleep. DSIP has also shown promise in improving resilience to stress-related sleep disturbances.

Another key compound is Epitalon, a tetrapeptide known for its role in regulating melatonin production. By acting on the pineal gland and resetting the circadian rhythm, Epitalon can normalize sleep-wake cycles, making it highly effective for individuals with disrupted sleep patterns, jet lag, or age-related declines in melatonin output. Consistent Epitalon use has also been associated with improved REM stability and total sleep time, especially in older adults.

GHRP-6, a growth hormone-releasing peptide, contributes indirectly to sleep enhancement through its stimulation of natural growth hormone (GH) secretion. Since GH release is tightly linked to deep sleep—particularly in the early part of the night—peptides that increase GH availability may enhance slow-wave sleep and physical recovery. GHRP-6 also influences hunger and stress hormones, which can impact nocturnal rest when unbalanced.

Together, these peptides create a biologically supportive environment for deeper, more restorative sleep, improving everything from cognitive clarity and emotional regulation to tissue regeneration and immune health.

However, peptides work best when paired with proper sleep hygiene. Factors such as consistent sleep and wake times, reduced screen exposure before bed, optimal room temperature, and reduced stimulant use are essential for maximizing peptide efficacy. Peptides do not override poor habits—they amplify existing conditions, whether beneficial or disruptive.

It's also essential to recognize that individual variability plays a major role. Some individuals may respond well to DSIP but not to GHRP-6, or vice versa. Dosing, timing, and cycle length should be tailored based on goals and monitored responses, ideally with input from a qualified healthcare professional.

When used responsibly, peptides like DSIP, Epitalon, and GHRP-6 offer targeted support for those seeking to improve sleep depth, regularity, and recovery quality. As we explore further, we'll examine how these and other sleep-enhancing peptides fit into a comprehensive strategy for circadian health and long-term performance.

Regulating Cortisol, Melatonin, and Recovery Cycles

Effective sleep optimization hinges on the delicate orchestration of key hormones—cortisol, melatonin, and growth hormone—which together shape the sleep-wake rhythm, influence emotional resilience, and govern the body's ability to repair and restore. When these cycles fall out of sync, sleep quality and daytime function decline. Peptides, through their ability to modulate endocrine and circadian signals, offer targeted support for restoring hormonal balance and enhancing recovery.

Cortisol, often labeled the "stress hormone," follows a diurnal curve, rising sharply in the early morning to promote alertness and energy, then tapering gradually as the day progresses. However, chronic stress, poor nutrition, and disrupted circadian rhythms can cause cortisol to remain elevated in the evening—interfering with sleep onset and suppressing melatonin. Peptides such as GHRP-2 and GHRP-6, while primarily growth hormone secretagogues, also influence corticotropin-releasing hormone (CRH) and the HPA axis, potentially helping to rebalance cortisol output and support a healthier rise-fall rhythm.

In contrast, melatonin serves as the primary signal for sleep initiation. It is secreted in response to darkness by the pineal gland and aligns the body's biological clock with the external environment. Artificial light exposure—especially blue light from screens—can suppress melatonin synthesis, leading to delayed sleep onset and poor sleep continuity. Epitalon, a synthetic pineal peptide, has been shown to regulate melatonin rhythms and restore circadian alignment, particularly in individuals experiencing jet lag, shift work fatigue, or age-related declines in melatonin production.

During deep, non-REM sleep, the body transitions into recovery mode—a phase marked by growth hormone release, tissue regeneration, and cellular repair. Peptides such as CJC-1295 and Ipamorelin optimize this recovery process by enhancing natural GH pulses without overstimulation of stress hormones. This supports muscle repair, metabolic reset, immune modulation, and cognitive restoration—hallmarks of high-quality, restorative sleep.

Together, this peptide-based strategy addresses the triad of sleep regulation:

- Reducing evening cortisol to quiet the mind and body
- Increasing melatonin production for smoother sleep initiation
- Enhancing recovery cycles to promote deep physiological restoration

However, hormonal balance cannot be outsourced to peptides alone. Sleep hygiene—structured routines, consistent bed and wake times, reduction of stimulants, light management, and emotional regulation—provides the foundation for all biological interventions to take effect. Peptides should be integrated strategically and cyclically, complementing—not compensating for—core lifestyle habits.

Each individual's hormonal and circadian blueprint is different. What restores balance in one person may create imbalance in another. Peptides must be personalized, monitored, and adjusted to suit unique recovery needs, training intensity, stress load, and overall health status.

Used appropriately, peptides such as Epitalon, GHRP-2, GHRP-6, CJC-1295, and Ipamorelin offer a refined means to realign the body's rhythms, restore hormonal harmony, and enhance both sleep quality and physical regeneration. As we continue our exploration, we'll look at how these peptides can be woven into broader recovery strategies that support sustainable energy, cognitive clarity, and long-term circadian health.

Nighttime Repair and Growth Hormone Support

Sleep is the body's prime window for deep repair, regeneration, and hormone cycling. During this time, especially in the early stages of non-REM sleep, the body secretes pulses of growth hormone (GH)—a vital anabolic signal that initiates tissue healing, muscle repair, fat metabolism, and cellular rejuvenation. Peptides that amplify or mimic this natural process can significantly enhance the benefits of sleep, helping optimize recovery, physique, and long-term wellness.

Growth hormone follows a strong circadian rhythm, with its highest surge typically occurring within the first 90 minutes of sleep—during slow-wave sleep (SWS). This timing is critical: if sleep is delayed, fragmented, or too short, the window for optimal GH release narrows, undermining the repair cycle and impairing recovery.

Peptides such as GHRP-2, GHRP-6, CJC-1295, and Ipamorelin work by stimulating the hypothalamus and pituitary to increase endogenous GH secretion, without the need for exogenous hormone replacement. These compounds mimic ghrelin or enhance GHRH signaling, leading to enhanced GH release that aligns with the body's natural rhythm.

- CJC-1295 extends the half-life of growth hormone-releasing hormone (GHRH), allowing for sustained GH release throughout the night.
- Ipamorelin is highly selective and doesn't raise cortisol or prolactin, making it ideal for nighttime use when hormonal balance is delicate.
- GHRP-2 and GHRP-6, while slightly more stimulatory, can provide potent GH pulses when used strategically.

When stacked appropriately—such as CJC-1295 with Ipamorelin—these peptides can significantly amplify nighttime repair cycles, supporting muscular recovery, fat oxidation, immune activity, and even neurological reset.

Another important sleep-specific peptide is DSIP (Delta Sleep-Inducing Peptide). Rather than directly stimulating GH, DSIP improves the depth and stability of delta-wave sleep, the stage most closely linked with GH secretion. By promoting deeper restorative sleep, DSIP indirectly supports stronger, more consistent nighttime GH release and improves recovery outcomes.

Together, these peptides create an internal environment that prioritizes recovery, regeneration, and metabolic recalibration during sleep.

However, the effectiveness of these peptides depends entirely on foundational sleep hygiene. Without a consistent bedtime, a dark and quiet environment, and avoidance of late-night stimulants and screen exposure, even the most potent peptides will fall short. Peptides amplify biological processes—they don't override poor behavioral patterns.

Additionally, individual responses vary. Personalized dosing, timing, and cycling are essential to avoid receptor desensitization or hormonal disruption. Any peptide-based regimen should be monitored by a practitioner experienced in peptide and circadian biology.

When used intelligently and integrated with strong lifestyle habits, peptides such as CJC-1295, Ipamorelin, GHRP-2, GHRP-6, and DSIP offer precise support for enhancing sleep quality, deepening recovery, and optimizing nightly growth hormone release. This combination forms the backbone of true overnight repair, helping ensure the body wakes restored, rebalanced, and ready to perform.

As our peptide journey continues, we'll explore how this nighttime optimization strategy fits into broader protocols for energy, cognitive resilience, and long-term hormonal health.

Building a Rest-Focused Peptide Protocol

Creating an effective peptide protocol for sleep and recovery begins with intention. Rather than adopting a one-size-fits-all approach, a rest-focused peptide strategy should align with your specific physiological goals—whether it's improving sleep depth, boosting nighttime growth hormone (GH) release, or accelerating post-training recovery. When thoughtfully assembled, such a protocol can enhance nightly restoration and elevate long-term performance.

Step 1: Define Your Objective

Begin by clearly identifying your primary outcome:

- Is your focus on improving sleep quality—falling asleep faster, sleeping deeper, and waking more refreshed?
- Are you prioritizing muscle repair, fat metabolism, or immune recovery during the night?
- Do you experience circadian misalignment, jet lag, or irregular sleep-wake patterns?

Your answer will guide your peptide selection and how you structure the protocol.

Step 2: Select the Appropriate Peptides

For deep, restorative sleep:

- DSIP (Delta Sleep-Inducing Peptide) — supports delta wave sleep and enhances sleep continuity
- Epitalon — regulates melatonin, reinforces circadian rhythm, and improves sleep regularity

For nighttime recovery and GH release:

- CJC-1295 — extends natural GHRH activity for prolonged GH release
- Ipamorelin — triggers GH pulses with minimal side effects, ideal for nighttime use
- GHRP-2 or GHRP-6 — strong GH secretagogues that may also modulate cortisol (better suited for earlier evening use due to appetite stimulation potential)

Step 3: Optimize Dosing and Timing

Peptides should be administered at times that align with natural hormonal rhythms.

- GH-releasing peptides are best used 30–60 minutes before sleep, ideally on an empty stomach to avoid insulin interference.
- DSIP or Epitalon can be administered just before bed, helping initiate deep sleep and regulate the internal clock.
- Start with minimal effective doses and increase cautiously. Titrate based on results and feedback from your body or clinician oversight.

Step 4: Anchor the Protocol with Strong Sleep Hygiene

Peptides are enhancers—not replacements—for foundational habits. To amplify effectiveness:

- Maintain consistent sleep and wake times, even on weekends
- Avoid bright light and screens for 1–2 hours before bed
- Create a dark, cool, and quiet sleep environment
- Limit stimulants (caffeine, nicotine) in the afternoon
- Reduce stress and late-night training, both of which elevate cortisol and disrupt GH rhythms

Step 5: Monitor and Adjust

Track your sleep quality, recovery, and energy levels using tools like sleep journals, HRV trackers, or wearable sleep devices. Adjust peptide combinations, timing, and dosing in response to trends. If a peptide causes vivid dreams, disrupted sleep, or fatigue, it may be mistimed or dosed too high.

Step 6: Work with a Healthcare Provider

Collaborating with a knowledgeable peptide-literate clinician ensures safety, efficacy, and regulatory compliance. They can also help determine when to cycle off peptides to avoid desensitization or hormonal imbalance.

When built strategically, a rest-focused peptide protocol offers precision support for deeper sleep, better hormone rhythm, and enhanced overnight regeneration. By aligning the right compounds with sound sleep habits, you amplify the body's ability to repair, grow, and perform—all while you rest.

As we continue this exploration, we'll dive into long-term strategies for cycling, combining, and customizing peptide use for ongoing circadian health and high-level recovery.

CHAPTER 6

MENTAL CLARITY AND MOOD REGULATION

Cognitive Peptides and Their Neurological Effects

Optimizing brain health is essential for sustaining cognitive performance, emotional balance, and mental endurance. The brain, governed by intricate biochemical signaling, requires support not only through lifestyle but also, potentially, through compounds designed to target specific neural mechanisms. Among these, certain peptides—referred to as cognitive peptides—demonstrate the ability to influence neural activity, enhance mental clarity, and improve mood regulation through direct interaction with the central nervous system.

Semax, Selank, and Noopept are among the most widely studied peptides for cognitive enhancement. Each acts through distinct pathways while producing measurable neurological effects. These include modulation of neurotransmitter systems, stimulation of neurotrophic factors, and regulation of neuroimmune responses, all of which impact cognition and emotional processing.

Semax increases expression of brain-derived neurotrophic factor (BDNF), a critical protein involved in synaptic repair, memory consolidation, and adaptive learning. Elevated BDNF levels support neural growth and plasticity, facilitating improved mental focus and emotional resilience. Semax also affects dopaminergic and serotonergic systems, further supporting executive function and stable mood.

Selank, derived from the naturally occurring immune modulator tuftsin, influences neurochemical stability by regulating the release and reuptake of serotonin and dopamine. This modulation can reduce anxiety, support calm focus, and promote cognitive flexibility. Additionally, Selank exhibits neuroprotective properties by dampening excessive inflammation within the brain, a contributor to mood disorders and cognitive dysfunction.

Noopept operates on glutamatergic pathways and stimulates production of both BDNF and nerve growth factor (NGF). These neurotrophins are key to maintaining the integrity of neuronal networks. Noopept may also enhance acetylcholine sensitivity and improve dopaminergic signaling, offering support for memory encoding, mental sharpness, and motivation.

These peptides function as part of a broader system, not as replacements for foundational cognitive health practices. Nutrition, sleep hygiene, physical movement, stress regulation, and neurostimulation (such as learning or creative engagement) remain essential. Peptides amplify physiological processes already in motion; they are not effective in isolation from supportive routines.

Clinical use of cognitive peptides is still expanding. While the available research indicates beneficial outcomes, long-term safety profiles and comparative efficacy are not yet fully established. Individual responses vary based on neurological baselines, dosage sensitivity, and preexisting conditions. Adjustments in dosage, frequency, or peptide combinations may be necessary depending on observed cognitive and emotional effects.

Monitoring changes in focus, processing speed, mental stamina, and mood variability can help guide protocol refinement. Professional supervision ensures peptide use remains safe, effective, and well-integrated with other interventions or medications.

Cognitive peptides such as Semax, Selank, and Noopept show potential in enhancing mental performance, stabilizing mood, and promoting long-term neurological health. Their mechanisms reflect a growing understanding of how targeted molecules can interface with brain function to support clarity, resilience, and adaptability in dynamic environments.

Supporting Focus, Memory, and Executive Function

Cognitive performance relies on the brain's ability to sustain attention, process and retain information, and manage complex tasks through coordinated executive function. These abilities underpin daily productivity, decision-making, and adaptive learning. Several peptides have shown promise in enhancing these specific domains by influencing neurochemical signaling, promoting synaptic plasticity, and supporting long-term potentiation.

Noopept is one of the most studied cognitive-enhancing peptides. It modulates the brain's glutamatergic system and elevates expression of brain-derived neurotrophic factor (BDNF), a protein critical for synaptic integrity and memory formation. Increased BDNF supports the survival of neurons and strengthens the neural circuits involved in learning and recall. Noopept's additional effects on acetylcholine sensitivity and dopaminergic tone contribute to heightened alertness and improved mental clarity.

Semax, another cognitive peptide, also stimulates BDNF while modulating key neurotransmitters such as dopamine and serotonin. These neuromodulators play a direct role in motivation, mood regulation, and cognitive processing. By enhancing their availability, Semax may increase sustained attention, improve short-term memory performance, and facilitate complex thought integration.

P21, a synthetic derivative of Cerebrolysin, acts on mechanisms associated with long-term potentiation (LTP)-a key process for encoding and stabilizing new memories. By supporting synaptic reinforcement and neurogenesis, P21 may aid in the retention and application of newly acquired knowledge, especially in contexts requiring prolonged cognitive demand or neurorestoration.

Collectively, these peptides influence multiple layers of brain function:

- BDNF and NGF enhancement to facilitate synaptic plasticity
- Neurotransmitter balance across dopaminergic, serotonergic, and glutamatergic pathways
- Support for LTP, enabling durable memory formation and efficient information retrieval

These mechanisms provide meaningful support for enhancing cognitive workload tolerance, increasing task-switching efficiency, and improving executive oversight.

However, peptide use should be approached as one element of a larger neurocognitive protocol. Sustained cognitive performance is shaped by cumulative lifestyle inputs-nutrient sufficiency, sleep architecture, circadian alignment, physical movement, stress adaptation, and cognitive stimulation. Peptides offer augmentation of these efforts, not substitution.

Responsiveness to cognitive peptides varies widely across individuals due to differences in baseline neurotransmitter profiles, genetic predispositions, and environmental stress loads. Therefore, gradual dosing, consistent tracking, and periodic reassessment are essential for optimizing results and minimizing potential overactivation or tolerance.

Clinician guidance ensures precision in compound selection, appropriate dosing intervals, and integration with other therapeutic strategies or nootropic regimens. Protocol customization may involve cycling peptides, combining them strategically, or rotating based on cognitive stress demands.

When used with intent and supported by a robust lifestyle foundation, peptides such as Noopept, Semax, and P21 can enhance focus, working memory, and executive function. Their targeted mechanisms align with the neurological underpinnings of peak cognitive output, offering a valuable set of tools for maintaining mental performance across high-demand contexts.

Combating Anxiety, Brain Fog, and Low Motivation

Cognitive strain, emotional volatility, and lack of drive are increasingly prevalent in modern life. High stress loads, environmental overstimulation, and fragmented routines contribute to persistent anxiety, reduced mental clarity, and motivational fatigue. Addressing these symptoms requires a multifaceted strategy-and certain peptides have emerged as tools capable of targeting the neurochemical imbalances that underlie these states.

Selank is a synthetic peptide with notable anxiolytic properties. It influences serotonin and dopamine metabolism, stabilizing mood and dampening hyperactive neural patterns without sedation. By supporting balanced neurotransmission, Selank helps regulate emotional tone, reduce reactivity, and promote mental clarity under stress. Its immunomodulatory properties may also support neuroimmune balance, which is often disrupted in chronic anxiety states.

Semax, sharing pharmacological overlap with Selank, also modulates serotonin and dopamine systems while simultaneously increasing brain-derived neurotrophic factor (BDNF) levels. BDNF enhances neuroplasticity and cognitive resilience, particularly in regions tied to memory and attention. By improving signal transmission and adaptive capacity, Semax offers dual-action benefits-easing anxiety while lifting mental fog and enhancing cognitive tempo.

Noopept targets dopaminergic reward pathways, enhancing motivation, drive, and task engagement. It facilitates neurochemical activation of the prefrontal cortex, where executive motivation originates. This peptide also boosts BDNF and NGF expression, which can improve working memory and mood stability during periods of low energy or mental disengagement.

These peptides support key neurochemical mechanisms:

- Dopamine enhancement for reward, drive, and cognitive momentum
- Serotonin regulation to stabilize emotional tone and reduce anxiety sensitivity
- BDNF stimulation for improved mental clarity, attention, and stress buffering

Their use is best positioned within a comprehensive mental health framework. Diet, circadian alignment, exercise, social support, and cognitive engagement remain the foundation for long-term mental stability. Peptides are tools for recalibrating neurochemical rhythm but must be layered onto sustainable behavioral practices.

Individual variability in neurotransmitter function and stress resilience means that responses to peptides like Selank, Semax, and Noopept will differ. Gradual titration, journaling cognitive or emotional shifts, and scheduled re-evaluations are essential to calibrate their use effectively.

Medical oversight ensures peptides are sourced reliably, dosed appropriately, and integrated safely alongside other supplements or medications. Clinical context also helps identify when deeper issues-such as hormonal dysregulation or inflammation-might underlie persistent symptoms.

By modulating the neurochemical systems responsible for anxiety control, cognitive engagement, and emotional regulation, peptides such as Selank, Semax, and Noopept offer targeted support for mental resilience. Their actions complement structural habits and may assist individuals in regaining clarity, motivation, and a stable internal rhythm during periods of strain or burnout.

Neuroprotective Potential of Select Peptides

Preserving brain health is a foundational goal in cognitive longevity and emotional stability. The central nervous system is vulnerable to cumulative damage from oxidative stress, neuroinflammation, and age-related degeneration. Certain peptides exhibit neuroprotective properties that may counteract these effects, supporting cellular integrity, slowing neuronal decline, and reinforcing resilience in vulnerable brain regions.

Cerebrolysin, a complex of low molecular weight peptides derived from porcine brain tissue, is one of the most studied agents in this category. It demonstrates the ability to reduce oxidative damage, excitotoxicity, and inflammatory signaling in neuronal tissues. By modulating apoptosis pathways and enhancing neurotrophic activity, Cerebrolysin supports neuronal survival and function under stress. It has been investigated in the context of traumatic brain injury, stroke recovery, and cognitive decline associated with aging and neurodegeneration.

Semax, while primarily known for its cognitive-enhancing effects, also exhibits robust neuroprotective activity. It upregulates brain-derived neurotrophic factor (BDNF) and modulates neuroimmune responses, two mechanisms essential for defending against structural and chemical insults to the brain. BDNF supports neuronal repair, synaptogenesis, and long-term resilience under cognitive or emotional load. By maintaining neurotrophic balance, Semax may mitigate degradation of cognitive processing over time.

P21, a synthetic analog inspired by Cerebrolysin, has gained interest for its ability to enhance long-term potentiation (LTP) and support synaptic memory encoding. Its neuroprotective effects are believed to stem from preservation of hippocampal activity and stimulation of signaling pathways involved in neural plasticity and regeneration. P21 may provide benefits in both preventative and restorative neurological contexts, particularly where memory and learning pathways are compromised.

The mechanisms through which these peptides act include:

- Inhibition of pro-inflammatory cytokines and oxidative enzymes
- Activation of neurotrophic cascades supporting neuronal survival and plasticity
- Stabilization of mitochondrial function and synaptic signaling
- Modulation of apoptosis and glutamate excitotoxicity, key contributors to neural cell loss

While promising, the use of neuroprotective peptides should complement—not replace—lifestyle practices that form the foundation of brain preservation. Regular aerobic movement, a polyphenol-rich diet, deep sleep cycles, and engagement in mentally stimulating activities form the physiological environment in which peptides exert optimal benefits.

Responses to peptide-based neuroprotection vary depending on age, existing neurological load, metabolic health, and genetic predispositions. Tracking cognitive markers, mood stability, and recovery patterns is key to assessing peptide effectiveness. Adjustments in timing or dosing may be necessary depending on neurological demand or phase of cognitive recovery.

Professional guidance ensures that peptide use is harmonized with other interventions, medications, or neurological therapies. Careful selection based on symptom profile, cognitive goals, and tolerance ensures these compounds deliver value without unintended overstimulation or metabolic disruption.

Peptides such as Cerebrolysin, Semax, and P21 offer potential protection against the progressive insults of inflammation, oxidative stress, and neural disconnection. Their integration into cognitive health protocols may extend functional mental capacity, buffer against decline, and preserve quality of thought across longer lifespans.

Optimizing Brain Chemistry Naturally

Neurochemical balance is central to mental clarity, emotional regulation, and sustained cognitive performance. The brain operates through a dynamic network of neurotransmitters and signaling molecules that influence thought processing, memory consolidation, motivation, and mood. While lifestyle factors remain the foundation for optimizing brain chemistry, certain peptides can provide targeted modulation of neurotransmitter systems and enhance the brain's natural equilibrium.

Semax and Selank are among the most effective peptides for supporting neurochemical regulation. These compounds interact with dopaminergic and serotonergic pathways, adjusting synaptic tone without overstimulation. By supporting dopamine availability, they promote drive, focus, and goal-directed behavior. Through modulation of serotonin, they contribute to emotional stability, reduced anxiety reactivity, and improved adaptability to stress.

Noopept extends neurochemical support through a broader spectrum. It influences acetylcholine, essential for attention and short-term memory, while also affecting glutamate, the brain's primary excitatory neurotransmitter. These interactions improve working memory, enhance mental agility, and support mood regulation through dopaminergic reinforcement.

The combined effects of these peptides include:

- Enhanced neurotransmitter efficiency, without creating excessive stimulation or rebound
- Improved neural communication across mood and cognition centers
- Greater resilience to stress-related dysregulation, aiding both performance and emotional control

Although these peptides assist in stabilizing brain chemistry, long-term mental health depends on broader inputs. Neurochemical balance is highly sensitive to circadian rhythm, micronutrient intake, physical activity, and recovery cycles. A stable foundation of sleep, nutrient diversity, and movement enables peptides to exert maximal benefit.

Biochemical individuality influences peptide efficacy. Variables such as preexisting neurotransmitter imbalances, genetic methylation profiles, or metabolic health can shape how a person responds to Semax, Selank, or Noopept. Incremental protocol adjustments based on mood tracking, cognitive shifts, or sleep quality can guide effective titration.

Medical oversight supports safe and effective use. It allows for fine-tuning of peptide selection, ensures compatibility with other cognitive or psychiatric therapies, and minimizes the risk of imbalances from long-term use. Responsible cycling and biomarker feedback are critical for sustaining gains without disrupting endogenous neurotransmission.

Peptides such as Semax, Selank, and Noopept serve as strategic tools for enhancing mental acuity, focus, and emotional steadiness. Their ability to modulate key neurotransmitters without overstimulation makes them suitable for both high-performance contexts and cognitive support under stress. Integrated into a broader strategy of brain health, these compounds can reinforce the body's innate capacity to maintain neurochemical harmony.

CHAPTER 7

HORMONAL BALANCE AND VITALITY

How Peptides Influence the Endocrine System

Hormones govern a wide array of vital functions—regulating metabolism, mood, energy, sexual function, and growth. This complex system, managed by the endocrine glands, relies on tightly controlled chemical signals. Select peptides can interact with these systems directly, acting on endocrine receptors or stimulating hormone production to support more balanced physiology and improved vitality.

Peptides operate as targeted messengers. Due to their structure, they can bind to specific receptors and modulate hormonal output through precise biochemical signaling. This ability allows them to influence major axes of the endocrine system, including growth, reproductive, and stress pathways.

Key examples of endocrine-targeting peptides include:

Growth Hormone Releasing Peptides (GHRPs)

- Examples: GHRP-2, GHRP-6, Ipamorelin
- Mechanism: Stimulate the anterior pituitary to increase growth hormone (GH) secretion
- Benefits: Enhanced lean muscle growth, fat metabolism, tissue repair, and overall rejuvenation

Gonadotropin-Releasing Hormone (GnRH) Analogues

- Examples: Triptorelin, Gonadorelin

- Mechanism: Act on the hypothalamus to regulate the release of luteinizing hormone (LH) and follicle-stimulating hormone (FSH)
- Benefits: Support testosterone and estrogen balance, improve reproductive health, and help modulate libido

HPA Axis Modulators

- Examples: Selank, Semax
- Mechanism: Normalize the feedback loops of the hypothalamic-pituitary-adrenal axis
- Benefits: Reduce cortisol dysregulation, promote calm focus, and sustain energy during high stress

These peptides act by restoring signaling balance across hormonal networks, rather than artificially replacing hormones. This indirect stimulation encourages the body to recalibrate its own production pathways, supporting more sustainable hormonal vitality.

Nonetheless, hormonal balance is governed by broader influences: nutrient status, circadian rhythm, body composition, and even environmental endocrine disruptors. Peptides offer precision within this system, but only in coordination with these foundational pillars.

Individual variation is significant. Peptide responses depend on age, baseline hormone levels, metabolic function, and preexisting glandular stress. Monitoring hormonal markers—such as free testosterone, IGF-1, cortisol rhythm, or FSH/LH ratios—is essential for tailoring peptide protocols effectively.

Clinical supervision remains critical. Practitioners trained in integrative endocrinology can assess your current status, recommend appropriate peptides, adjust dosing protocols, and ensure alignment with any existing hormone therapies or medical conditions.

Peptides such as GHRPs, GnRH analogues, and HPA modulators demonstrate measurable potential to restore hormonal vitality by stimulating natural endocrine rhythms. They offer a functional approach to correcting subtle imbalances that, over time, degrade energy, resilience, and well-being. Used wisely and within a structured plan, they can enhance the body's capacity to maintain hormonal health across the lifespan.

Supporting Testosterone, Growth Hormone, and Libido

Testosterone, growth hormone, and libido form a tightly interconnected triad that influences strength, energy, metabolism, and sexual vitality. When these systems function optimally, they support physical performance, emotional resilience, and overall quality of life. Peptides offer a means of supporting these hormones by working with the body's own regulatory pathways rather than overriding them.

Testosterone, produced predominantly in the testes in men and in smaller amounts by the ovaries and adrenal glands in women, is essential for maintaining muscle mass, bone density, mood stability, and sexual health. One peptide that can influence testosterone indirectly is Gonadorelin. It mimics the action of gonadotropin-releasing hormone, prompting the pituitary to secrete luteinizing hormone (LH) and follicle-stimulating hormone (FSH). These hormones stimulate the testes to produce testosterone. This upstream stimulation supports natural testosterone production and helps maintain balanced endocrine function without suppressing feedback mechanisms.

Growth hormone, secreted by the anterior pituitary, governs lean tissue development, recovery, fat metabolism, and overall regenerative capacity. It also plays a critical role in maintaining youth-associated physiological traits. Growth hormone-releasing peptides, including GHRP-2, GHRP-6, and Ipamorelin, are frequently used to enhance endogenous GH output. These peptides increase the frequency and amplitude of GH pulses, which can lead to increased production of IGF-1, a key driver of muscle repair and cellular regeneration. This enhanced hormonal environment supports lean muscle growth, fat oxidation, better sleep quality, and higher overall energy levels.

Libido, or sexual desire, reflects a dynamic interplay between hormonal levels, neurological inputs, and psychological state. While testosterone is a major factor, central nervous system activity also plays a vital role. PT-141, also known as Bremelanotide, offers a novel mechanism of action. Rather than acting on blood flow like traditional erectile dysfunction medications, PT-141 works through melanocortin receptor activation in the brain. This central action has been associated with heightened sexual arousal and increased responsiveness to stimuli, in both men and women. Its use is particularly notable in cases where libido is suppressed despite otherwise normal hormone levels.

Although these peptides have shown measurable benefits in clinical and anecdotal settings, they are not substitutes for foundational health practices. Nutrition, physical training, recovery, sleep quality, and stress regulation each contribute directly to hormonal regulation and sexual function. Peptides should be viewed as part of a broader lifestyle framework rather than standalone interventions.

Hormonal variability between individuals means that even well-targeted peptides may produce different outcomes from one person to the next. Lab testing, symptom tracking, and expert guidance are essential to tailoring peptide use to individual needs. This is especially important when working with hormones that affect reproductive and metabolic systems.

Under the supervision of an experienced healthcare provider, peptides like Gonadorelin, the GHRP family, and PT-141 can serve as effective tools for enhancing testosterone, growth hormone, and libido. They offer a more naturalistic approach by encouraging the body to regulate itself, rather than imposing synthetic hormone levels from the outside. When integrated into a responsible and well-structured protocol, they can contribute meaningfully to restored hormonal health and long-term vitality.

Women's Health Considerations

Hormonal balance in women is governed by a finely tuned interplay of estrogen, progesterone, testosterone, and other regulatory signals that shift over time and across life stages. These fluctuations not only shape reproductive function but also affect mood, metabolism, bone density, and tissue resilience. Peptides offer potential to support key aspects of this dynamic system through mechanisms that enhance or stabilize endocrine activity without overriding the body's internal feedback loops.

Kisspeptin-10 stands out for its critical role in reproductive signaling. It acts on the hypothalamus to initiate the release of gonadotropin-releasing hormone (GnRH), which in turn stimulates the secretion of luteinizing hormone (LH) and follicle-stimulating hormone (FSH). These hormones are essential for regulating ovulation and menstrual cyclicity. In women experiencing irregular cycles, diminished ovarian response, or fertility challenges, Kisspeptin-10 may help restore hormonal communication and support ovarian function by promoting a synchronized GnRH pulse.

Thymosin Beta-4 (TB-4) demonstrates a different kind of benefit. Its anti-inflammatory properties have drawn attention for managing gynecological conditions involving chronic inflammation, such as endometriosis. By modulating the inflammatory response, TB-4 may help alleviate pelvic pain and reduce the progression of lesions associated with abnormal endometrial tissue growth. Its wound-healing and immune-modulatory effects offer additional value in systemic recovery and post-surgical healing scenarios common to women's health care.

Peptides that stimulate growth hormone secretion—namely GHRP-2, GHRP-6, and Ipamorelin—can also support women's hormonal balance by promoting metabolic stability, muscle preservation, and bone density. Growth hormone naturally declines with age, and this decline contributes to muscle loss, insulin resistance, and fragility. These peptides enhance the body's own pulsatile release of growth hormone, potentially improving recovery, lean mass retention, and overall energy metabolism without introducing exogenous hormones.

It is essential to recognize that hormonal symptoms in women—ranging from fatigue and low libido to cycle irregularity and mood shifts—are rarely caused by a single factor. Endocrine health is affected by nutrition, sleep quality, stress load, gut health, and environmental exposures. Peptide protocols are most effective when combined with comprehensive strategies that address these foundational elements. Lifestyle alignment remains a critical variable in whether peptide-based interventions deliver sustainable benefits.

Responses to peptides are highly individualized. Genetic variation, hormonal history, and current metabolic status all influence peptide efficacy and tolerance. Close monitoring, regular lab assessments, and clear outcome tracking help refine protocols and reduce the likelihood of unwanted effects.

Before initiating any peptide therapy, consultation with a provider who understands endocrine signaling, peptide pharmacodynamics, and personalized dosing strategies is non-negotiable. Professional oversight ensures that therapies are not only safe but also aligned with evolving needs and hormonal feedback patterns.

Peptides such as Kisspeptin-10, TB-4, and the GHRP class represent promising tools for supporting hormonal health in women. When used with precision and paired with strong foundational health practices, they can help stabilize hormone rhythms, enhance reproductive wellness, and strengthen the systems that underpin long-term vitality.

Peptides and the HPA Axis

The Hypothalamic-Pituitary-Adrenal (HPA) axis orchestrates the body's central response to stress. This neuroendocrine network links the hypothalamus, pituitary gland, and adrenal glands in a cascade of hormonal signaling that influences digestion, immunity, mood regulation, reproductive function, and energy balance. Disruptions in this axis can lead to chronic stress patterns, fatigue, mood instability, and metabolic dysfunction. Select peptides offer the potential to modulate the HPA axis with precision, influencing how the body adapts to both acute and long-term stressors.

Corticotropin-Releasing Factor (CRF) initiates the HPA stress response. It is secreted by the hypothalamus when a perceived stressor is detected. CRF then signals the pituitary gland to release adrenocorticotropic hormone (ACTH), which travels to the adrenal cortex and stimulates cortisol production. Elevated cortisol increases alertness and mobilizes energy stores but can also suppress immune function and impair recovery when chronically elevated. Peptides capable of modulating CRF activity may help recalibrate the HPA axis, reducing the burden of prolonged cortisol dominance and restoring homeostasis.

Vasopressin, also involved in HPA regulation, amplifies the ACTH-releasing effect of CRF during stress. It acts synergistically with CRF, intensifying the adrenal response. Peptides that influence vasopressin signaling could therefore fine-tune the magnitude and duration of the cortisol response, potentially improving recovery and reducing systemic wear from chronic activation.

Selank and Semax, synthetic peptides developed in Russia, demonstrate distinct effects on HPA axis modulation. Both compounds influence the balance of neurotransmitters and neurohormones involved in stress resilience. Selank has been observed to reduce anxiety-like behaviors in preclinical studies and may inhibit excessive CRF signaling. Semax enhances cognitive resilience and appears to support adaptive responses by promoting neurotrophic factors while also dampening stress-related overactivation. These peptides do not blunt the HPA axis entirely; rather, they help normalize its rhythm and restore adaptive range.

While these peptides offer targeted support for stress regulation, the HPA axis does not operate in isolation. It is shaped by lifestyle inputs such as circadian rhythm stability, nutritional sufficiency, glycemic control, and consistent physical activity. Chronic sleep deprivation, unresolved trauma, and persistent systemic inflammation can perpetuate maladaptive HPA patterns regardless of peptide support.

Individual variability must also be factored into any peptide-based approach. Baseline cortisol rhythm, adrenal function, psychological stress load, and neurochemical sensitivity differ from person to person. Peptide response may vary depending on whether the individual is dealing with burnout, hypervigilance, trauma-related dysregulation, or general fatigue.

Healthcare supervision is essential. A qualified practitioner can assess HPA dysfunction through targeted lab work, interpret biomarker patterns, and guide peptide selection and dosing. Regular follow-up ensures peptides are titrated correctly, aligned with progress markers, and adjusted for emerging needs.

Peptides that interact with the HPA axis—such as CRF modulators, Vasopressin regulators, Selank, and Semax—may offer a refined strategy for enhancing stress resilience. By addressing the root hormonal architecture of the stress response, these peptides expand the toolkit for restoring vitality and rebalancing mood, energy, and emotional stability.

Smart Stacking for Hormonal Synergy

Combining peptides with complementary effects—known as smart stacking—can amplify physiological benefits by enhancing hormonal synergy. When thoughtfully designed, peptide stacks can optimize endocrine signaling, improve hormonal rhythms, and support broader vitality goals with greater precision than single-agent protocols.

A common synergistic pairing involves growth hormone-releasing peptides (GHRPs) like Ipamorelin and growth hormone-releasing hormones (GHRHs) such as CJC-1295. GHRPs directly stimulate the pituitary gland to release growth hormone. GHRHs, in contrast, suppress somatostatin, the hormone that inhibits growth hormone release. Stacking these together can significantly elevate growth hormone output, supporting lean muscle development, fat metabolism, tissue repair, and bone density.

Another effective combination targets both reproductive and sexual health. Kisspeptin-10 promotes the release of gonadotropin-releasing hormone (GnRH), supporting menstrual cycle regulation and fertility. PT-141, meanwhile, acts on melanocortin receptors in the brain to enhance sexual arousal. Used together, these peptides may address hormonal irregularities while boosting libido—an integrative approach to hormonal wellness.

Smart stacking can also be tailored to support adrenal balance and resilience. Selank and Semax, both of which modulate the hypothalamic-pituitary-adrenal (HPA) axis, can be paired with peptides like GHK-Cu for enhanced cognitive clarity, mood stabilization, and improved stress recovery. By aligning peptides with specific hormonal pathways and functional outcomes, the stack becomes more than the sum of its parts.

However, stacking must be individualized. Endocrine sensitivity, baseline hormone levels, age, lifestyle factors, and metabolic state all influence peptide response. An effective combination for one individual may yield suboptimal or counterproductive results for another.

Clinical oversight is essential. Hormonal stacks must be supported by lab testing, symptom tracking, and expert guidance. A healthcare provider can fine-tune dosages, cycle durations, and timing to match the user's evolving needs and minimize adverse effects or hormonal imbalances.

Peptide stacking strategies should also be anchored in foundational health principles. Nutrient density, glycemic control, circadian stability, restorative sleep, and regular exercise create the biological context in which peptides can exert their full benefits. Without these pillars, even a well-designed stack will have limited impact.

When constructed with insight and precision, peptide stacks can fine-tune hormonal outputs, restore rhythm to disrupted systems, and enhance the physiological coherence necessary for sustained vitality.

CHAPTER 8

IMMUNE RESILIENCE AND RECOVERY

Peptides That Support Immune Cell Function

The immune system operates as a sophisticated surveillance and defense network, composed of specialized cells and signaling mechanisms that detect and respond to pathogens, injury, and cellular abnormalities. Certain peptides enhance this system by modulating immune cell activity, increasing cellular communication, and accelerating recovery processes.

Thymosin Alpha-1 is one of the most well-researched immune-modulating peptides. Naturally secreted by the thymus, it enhances T cell maturation and responsiveness—key actions in both adaptive immunity and pathogen clearance. By upregulating T cell activity, Thymosin Alpha-1 reinforces the body's frontline immune defenses, particularly under chronic stress or during recovery from illness.

Thymosin Beta-4 complements this immune support by promoting tissue regeneration and modulating inflammation. It influences macrophage activation, supports lymphocyte signaling, and contributes to faster resolution of inflammatory responses. Its dual role in immune modulation and tissue repair makes it valuable for recovery from physical injury or immune exhaustion.

BPC-157, a peptide derived from gastric juice, supports immune health through its regulatory effects on gut integrity. Since a significant portion of the immune system resides in the gastrointestinal tract, maintaining gut barrier function is critical. BPC-157 aids in mucosal healing, reduces local inflammation, and fosters microbial balance—all essential to immune system competence.

Other peptides may indirectly support immune resilience by reducing systemic inflammation, enhancing antioxidant defenses, or supporting neuroendocrine pathways that impact immune coordination.

Still, peptides should be viewed as augmentative agents. Core immune function is shaped by nutritional status, circadian stability, microbial diversity, physical activity, and stress regulation. Peptides can amplify recovery and performance, but not replace foundational health practices.

Each person's immune profile, history of illness, and response to peptides will differ. Responsiveness may vary based on age, gut health, prior infections, or concurrent medication use. Protocols should be individualized and adapted over time.

A licensed practitioner can assist with dosage titration, safety monitoring, and lab evaluation to track immune markers. Supervised use ensures peptide interventions align with the user's physiology and current immune demands.

When used with strategic precision, peptides like Thymosin Alpha-1, Thymosin Beta-4, and BPC-157 can strengthen immune defense, accelerate healing, and enhance resilience in periods of stress or immune suppression.

Enhancing Resistance to Infections

The body's ability to defend against infections relies on a well-coordinated immune response capable of identifying, targeting, and neutralizing invading pathogens. Peptides that modulate immune pathways offer practical means to strengthen this defense, particularly in individuals facing immune suppression or heightened pathogen exposure.

Thymosin Alpha-1 is a thymic peptide that enhances T lymphocyte activation, central to adaptive immunity. T cells coordinate responses to viral and bacterial antigens, regulate other immune cells, and establish immunologic memory. By promoting T cell efficiency and activity, Thymosin Alpha-1 supports faster, more precise pathogen recognition and clearance. Its use has been studied extensively in viral infections and immune-compromised populations.

LL-37, an antimicrobial peptide derived from the cathelicidin family, exhibits direct bactericidal and antiviral activity. It disrupts microbial membranes, neutralizes endotoxins, and modulates inflammatory responses. LL-37 also enhances immune cell recruitment to infection sites, bridging innate and adaptive defenses. Its broad-spectrum efficacy makes it a potent adjunct in infection prevention strategies.

BPC-157, originally recognized for its gastrointestinal healing properties, also displays systemic immunomodulatory and antimicrobial effects. By supporting gut integrity, reducing local inflammation, and accelerating mucosal healing, BPC-157 indirectly reduces pathogen entry and strengthens barrier immunity. It may be especially relevant in maintaining resistance to gastrointestinal infections and restoring immune resilience following illness.

Peptides that support infection resistance are most effective when combined with foundational health strategies. These include micronutrient-rich diets, sleep optimization, physical conditioning, microbiome support, and inflammation control. Lifestyle patterns, stress exposure, and underlying medical conditions all influence infection susceptibility and should be addressed alongside peptide interventions.

Responses to immune peptides vary across individuals, shaped by genetic background, pathogen history, and immunological status. Personalized protocols are essential, particularly in cases of chronic illness, autoimmunity, or compromised immunity. Regular tracking of inflammatory markers, immune function, and infection outcomes can guide dose adjustments and peptide selection.

Healthcare supervision remains vital. Practitioners can tailor peptide combinations to fit real-time immune demands, ensure safety, and avoid counterproductive stimulation in autoimmune or overactive immune states.

When integrated appropriately, peptides like Thymosin Alpha-1, LL-37, and BPC-157 can strengthen host defense mechanisms, reduce infection risk, and support faster recovery from illness. Used in synergy with foundational health practices, they represent a dynamic addition to modern immune optimization.

Autoimmune and Inflammatory Considerations

Autoimmune diseases and chronic inflammation present major challenges to immune health. In these states, the body's defense system becomes dysregulated—either attacking healthy tissues or sustaining low-grade inflammatory responses that contribute to pain, fatigue, and tissue damage. Peptides with immunomodulatory and anti-inflammatory effects offer targeted options for helping restore immune balance and reduce symptom burden.

Thymosin Beta-4 (TB-4) has been noted for its role in downregulating pro-inflammatory cytokines and supporting tissue repair. In autoimmune conditions, where immune overactivity is common, TB-4 may help dampen the inappropriate activation of immune cells. By modulating the immune cascade and reducing systemic inflammation, it may also alleviate associated symptoms such as joint swelling, muscle soreness, and general fatigue.

BPC-157, derived from gastric proteins, offers dual action: regulating immune responses and healing gastrointestinal tissue. Since many autoimmune and inflammatory disorders involve compromised gut integrity—often referred to as "leaky gut"—BPC-157's ability to promote mucosal healing and reduce localized inflammation makes it especially relevant. This gut-centric benefit may indirectly reduce systemic autoimmune triggers and improve immune resilience.

Peptide interventions in autoimmune contexts require careful integration into broader treatment frameworks. Key strategies include reducing dietary triggers, managing oxidative stress, supporting adrenal function, optimizing sleep quality, and identifying environmental factors that drive inflammation. Peptides can enhance this foundation but should never be viewed as standalone solutions.

Because immune responses in autoimmune conditions are highly individualized, it is critical to monitor biomarkers of inflammation and immune function throughout any peptide regimen. Some patients may respond quickly, while others require longer durations or dose adjustments based on real-time feedback and clinical observation.

Medical oversight is essential. Healthcare professionals experienced in peptide therapeutics can help navigate potential interactions, minimize adverse effects, and fine-tune the protocol to reflect evolving symptoms or flare cycles.

Peptides like Thymosin Beta-4 and BPC-157 hold promise for reducing chronic inflammation and correcting immune dysfunction in autoimmune disease. Used thoughtfully within a personalized care plan, they offer a means of easing symptom load and supporting long-term immune recalibration.

Recovery from Illness and Physical Stress

The body's recovery process after illness or physical exertion is complex and deeply integrated with immune, metabolic, and regenerative systems. Peptides that support healing pathways can offer an edge in restoring balance and accelerating repair.

BPC-157, derived from gastric proteins, is well-studied for its regenerative effects. It appears to support mucosal integrity in the gastrointestinal tract, a region often compromised during chronic illness or systemic inflammation. By reinforcing the gut lining, BPC-157 can improve immune modulation and nutrient absorption—two factors critical for systemic recovery.

In physically stressed states, such as post-exertion fatigue or soft tissue injuries, BPC-157 may also assist in structural repair. It has demonstrated potential in accelerating tendon, ligament, and muscle healing, helping the body return to baseline more quickly after mechanical strain.

Thymosin Beta-4 (TB-4) is another peptide frequently cited for its anti-inflammatory and tissue-repairing effects. By downregulating pro-inflammatory cytokines and supporting cellular regeneration, TB-4 may ease pain and swelling while facilitating recovery in both infectious and injury-based stress states. Its role in angiogenesis and immune regulation makes it a particularly versatile option.

Successful recovery, however, depends on more than isolated biological triggers. Adequate nutrition, restorative sleep, and effective stress management are essential for peptides to work efficiently. Without these foundational supports, even the most targeted peptide intervention will deliver limited results.

Responses to peptide-based recovery protocols vary widely. Some individuals may experience rapid improvements, while others require tailored dosing strategies and extended use. Monitoring for progress and adapting as needed is key.

Professional oversight ensures proper integration into recovery plans. A healthcare provider familiar with peptide therapy can help refine timing, sequence, and combinations to match the body's evolving needs and healing cycles.

Peptides like BPC-157 and TB-4 offer valuable support in the recovery process, helping the body repair faster and more efficiently. Used strategically, they can complement a structured wellness plan and strengthen the body's natural ability to bounce back from stress or illness.

Safe Use in Immune-Modulating Protocols

Peptides can be powerful allies in supporting immune resilience, but their effectiveness depends on careful, informed use. Precision, personalization, and ongoing evaluation are essential to integrating peptides safely into immune-modulating protocols.

Every peptide operates on specific biological pathways. These effects vary widely depending on an individual's physiology, health status, and existing medications or supplements. What proves effective for one person may trigger adverse reactions in another. A foundational principle of safe use is individualization—monitoring responses closely and modifying protocols accordingly.

Proper dosing is critical. Peptides are biologically active at small concentrations, and increasing dosages without clinical rationale increases the risk of side effects. Common pitfalls include assuming that higher doses lead to quicker results or combining too many peptides without understanding their interactions. Safe use requires starting with the lowest effective dose and only adjusting under professional supervision.

Timing also matters. Some peptides exhibit diurnal patterns in their effectiveness—growth hormone-releasing peptides, for instance, may be more effective when administered in the evening. Others may interact differently with food, exercise, or concurrent therapies. Aligning peptide timing with the body's natural rhythms can significantly enhance their efficacy and tolerability.

No peptide should exist in a vacuum. Their benefits are maximized when integrated into a foundation of health that includes nutrient-dense meals, regular physical movement, restorative sleep, and effective stress regulation. Peptides can amplify these efforts, but they cannot replace them.

Working with a knowledgeable healthcare provider ensures correct selection, sequencing, and timing. Clinicians familiar with peptide pharmacodynamics can help you navigate contraindications, manage side effects, and measure progress with objective markers. This guidance is essential when immune function is being actively modulated.

Safe, strategic peptide use begins with awareness and ends with precision. A well-structured protocol, personalized to your physiology and guided by expertise, provides a path to enhanced immune support without unnecessary risk.

CHAPTER 9

DELIVERY METHODS AND DOSAGE PROTOCOLS

Injections vs. Oral vs. Nasal Spray vs. Topicals

The method by which a peptide is delivered plays a significant role in its effectiveness. Absorption rate, bioavailability, and site-specific action all depend on how the compound enters the body. Each delivery route offers distinct advantages and limitations, depending on the peptide's properties and intended use.

Injections remain the gold standard for peptide delivery, especially for systemic effects. Administered subcutaneously or intramuscularly, injections allow peptides to bypass the digestive system and enter directly into circulation. This results in high bioavailability and rapid onset. However, injections require sterile technique, precision in dosing, and comfort with needles—factors that can deter some users.

Oral delivery provides a more convenient and familiar method, especially for those averse to needles. The trade-off is a significant reduction in bioavailability. Enzymatic breakdown and first-pass metabolism in the liver degrade many peptides before they can exert their effects. Despite this, certain peptides—like BPC-157—demonstrate resilience in the gastrointestinal tract and remain biologically active when taken orally.

Nasal sprays offer a middle ground between oral and injectable options. The rich vascular network of the nasal mucosa enables rapid absorption into the bloodstream while avoiding the gastrointestinal tract. This route can be effective for smaller peptides or those targeting central nervous system effects. However, variability in absorption, potential irritation, and limited volume capacity make nasal delivery unsuitable for all peptides.

Topical formulations, including creams, gels, or patches, are primarily used for peptides targeting localized effects—most commonly in dermatology or joint care. When designed correctly, these formulations can penetrate the skin barrier and deliver active compounds to underlying tissues. However, inconsistent absorption and limited penetration depth can reduce efficacy.

The choice of delivery method should align with the specific peptide, desired outcome, and user preference. While injections remain the most efficient for systemic use, oral, nasal, and topical options expand accessibility and compliance for various health goals.

Delivery decisions should always be informed by the peptide's stability, absorption characteristics, and clinical purpose—guided by a practitioner familiar with peptide pharmacology.

How to Prepare and Administer Peptides Safely

Effective use of peptides begins with proper handling. Whether delivered via injection, oral supplement, nasal spray, or topical application, preparation and administration directly impact safety and bioavailability.

Injectable peptides typically arrive in lyophilized form and require reconstitution. Use bacteriostatic water to mix the powder into a solution, following exact concentration guidelines provided by the manufacturer. Reconstituted peptides must be refrigerated and shielded from light to preserve stability.

Sterile technique is non-negotiable. Always clean the injection site with alcohol, use a new sterile needle for each dose, and dispose of syringes in a sharps container. Subcutaneous injections are placed into the fatty layer beneath the skin, while intramuscular injections go deeper into the muscle. The appropriate method depends on the specific peptide and healthcare instructions.

Oral peptides, available in capsule or tablet form, are easier to administer but require consistency. Some are more effective on an empty stomach, while others may need to be taken with food. Follow dosing guidance carefully to optimize absorption.

Nasal sprays deliver peptides through the vascular nasal membrane. Lean your head back slightly, insert the spray tip into the nostril, and inhale gently while pressing the applicator. Avoid blowing your nose immediately after use. Be consistent with timing and dosage.

Topical peptides—gels, creams, or transdermal patches—should be applied to clean, dry skin. Rub in gently to aid absorption and prevent transfer to clothing or other surfaces. Avoid application to broken or irritated skin.

Across all formats, track your body's response. Redness, swelling, irritation, or digestive symptoms may indicate sensitivity or improper dosing. Pause use and consult a provider if adverse effects occur.

Peptides are potent tools, but safe use requires precision. Clean technique, correct dosing, and proper storage are essential for both effectiveness and safety. Always work in coordination with a knowledgeable healthcare provider.

Understanding Half-Lives, Timing, and Bioavailability

Effective use of peptides requires more than selecting the right compound—it demands a clear grasp of pharmacokinetics. Three critical elements shape how peptides perform in the body: half-life, timing, and bioavailability. Each plays a vital role in determining how often and when to administer a peptide, and how efficiently the body absorbs and utilizes it.

The half-life of a peptide defines how long it takes for its concentration in the bloodstream to be reduced by 50%. Peptides with short half-lives may require multiple doses per day to maintain therapeutic levels. Ipamorelin, for example, has a half-life of roughly two hours, often necessitating multiple daily injections. In contrast, CJC-1295 boasts a long half-life—about one week—allowing for weekly or biweekly administration.

Timing is equally important. Administering peptides in sync with the body's natural hormonal rhythms can enhance efficacy. Growth hormone-releasing peptides are often taken at night to coincide with peak nocturnal growth hormone pulses. Others may yield better absorption when timed around meals or physical activity. Some peptides, such as GHRPs, are best taken on an empty stomach, while others, like certain metabolic peptides, can be taken with food.

Bioavailability measures the fraction of a peptide that enters circulation and produces a biological effect. Delivery method heavily influences this. Injectables offer the highest bioavailability by bypassing digestive enzymes and liver metabolism. Oral peptides typically face more breakdown in the gastrointestinal tract, reducing their effectiveness. However, exceptions exist—BPC-157 demonstrates strong oral bioavailability despite being non-injectable.

Designing a peptide protocol requires aligning half-life, timing, and bioavailability with the user's goals and physiology. Metabolism, age, diet, and activity levels can all impact how a peptide performs in an individual. Adjustments should be based on observed outcomes rather than rigid schedules.

Work closely with a healthcare provider when determining dosing frequency and timing. Their oversight ensures the safest and most effective protocol, customized to your unique profile.

Understanding how peptides behave in the body is key to maximizing results and minimizing unnecessary dosing or inefficacy. The right strategy makes all the difference.

Protocol Lengths and Cycling Strategies

Developing an effective peptide regimen requires more than choosing the right compound—it involves structuring the duration of use and rest periods with precision. Protocol lengths and cycling strategies are essential for maximizing results while preserving safety, avoiding tolerance, and supporting long-term health.

Protocol length refers to how long a peptide is used in a given cycle. This can range from a few weeks to several months depending on the compound, the intended outcome, and the user's age, metabolic rate, baseline health, and lifestyle demands. Some peptides, particularly those that influence sleep or cognition, may yield results within weeks, while peptides aimed at body recomposition or hormonal support often require longer-term use.

Cycling is the practice of alternating between periods of use and intentional breaks. This strategy prevents receptor desensitization and maintains the peptide's effectiveness over time. It also allows the body to reset its baseline and avoid overstimulation of specific pathways. A widely adopted approach is 8 to 12 weeks on, followed by a 4 to 6-week break. This provides sufficient stimulation during the on-cycle and a physiological reset during the off-cycle.

Not all peptides require the same approach. Growth hormone secretagogues may benefit from longer use due to their gradual, compounding effects. Conversely, peptides used for acute goals—like injury recovery or immune modulation—may be applied in shorter, more targeted intervals.

Peptides often induce lasting physiological shifts. Enhanced growth hormone levels, better insulin sensitivity, or immune priming may persist beyond the final dose. For this reason, even off-cycle periods can bring continued benefits, further justifying strategic cycling.

Flexibility is key. Protocol design must account for the individual's response, progress, and any side effects. Overuse or continuous cycling without breaks can increase risks, reduce efficacy, and burden the endocrine system. Periodic reassessment is necessary.

Work with a qualified healthcare provider to determine appropriate durations, rest intervals, and transition strategies between cycles. This ensures you adapt your protocol safely and in alignment with your goals.

Well-structured protocol lengths and cycling strategies are not optional—they're foundational. With careful planning, you can avoid plateaus, enhance long-term results, and support sustainable peptide use across any area of focus.

Building a Routine That Fits Your Goals

Designing a peptide regimen begins with clarity about your personal goals. Whether your focus is muscle development, fat reduction, cognitive enhancement, or better sleep, aligning your protocol with those outcomes is essential for success.

Start by identifying your primary objective. Are you looking to accelerate recovery, support neuroplasticity, or improve hormonal balance? Defining this clearly enables targeted peptide selection.

Once your aim is established, choose compounds that are best suited to achieve it:

- For muscle growth or metabolic enhancement, peptides like CJC-1295 or Ipamorelin can support growth hormone release and body composition improvements.
- For sleep quality, DSIP is often favored for promoting deep, restorative sleep.
- For focus and mood regulation, Semax or Noopept may be more aligned with cognitive performance goals.

Peptide timing plays a critical role. Some compounds align better with specific circadian rhythms or metabolic states. Growth hormone secretagogues, for instance, are typically administered at night to match natural GH pulses. Others, like nootropic peptides, may be timed around periods of mental exertion.

Your protocol length and cycle design should reflect your goal's intensity and duration. A short-term goal like injury recovery might call for a few weeks of targeted use, while muscle-building or fat-loss protocols often benefit from longer durations, usually cycled with rest phases to prevent desensitization and maintain efficacy.

Each routine must remain adaptable. Monitor your response closely and adjust dosage, frequency, or combinations based on how your body reacts. Subtle tweaks can make a significant difference in overall results.

A peptide regimen works best when paired with foundational wellness practices. Nutrition, sleep hygiene, training, and stress control remain the cornerstones. Peptides are not a shortcut—they're a means to amplify your efforts when used strategically and responsibly.

Tailoring a routine to your objectives requires intention and attention. Start with a clear goal, match it with the right compounds, observe timing and cycling protocols, and support the process with healthy daily habits. With precision and consistency, peptides can become a highly effective tool in your personal optimization strategy.

CHAPTER 10
STACKING PEPTIDES WITH OTHER SUPPLEMENTS

Nutrients That Enhance Peptide Effectiveness

Pairing peptides with the right nutrients can improve absorption, enhance their physiological effects, and support the body's natural repair and regeneration systems. Strategic combinations offer an opportunity to reinforce peptide protocols with supplemental tools that help maximize results.

Peptides are composed of amino acids, making dietary protein a foundational component of any peptide-enhancing strategy. Sufficient protein intake ensures the body has the raw materials it needs for cellular repair, hormone production, and the synthesis of its own peptide hormones. Specific amino acids, like arginine, can further support peptide function by promoting the release of growth hormone when used alongside compounds such as CJC-1295 or Ipamorelin.

Vitamin C is another key nutrient for anyone using peptides that target skin, joint, or connective tissue health. Peptides like GHK-Cu, which stimulate collagen production, work more effectively when vitamin C levels are optimal, as this vitamin is essential for collagen synthesis.

Omega-3 fatty acids—found in fish oil, algae, and flaxseed—can complement the anti-inflammatory effects of regenerative peptides such as BPC-157 or TB-500. When recovering from injury, this combination may promote faster healing and reduced discomfort.

Adaptogens and herbal extracts can also amplify the benefits of peptide therapy. Ashwagandha, for example, may support natural growth hormone release and reduce cortisol, potentially improving outcomes when stacked with growth hormone secretagogues.

Electrolytes like magnesium and zinc should not be overlooked. Magnesium supports muscle recovery and nervous system function, while zinc is involved in hormone production and immune regulation—both of which can influence how the body responds to peptide signaling.

Despite the synergies, stacking should be approached thoughtfully. Supplements are not replacements for a well-rounded diet, and their effects vary based on individual biochemistry, age, health status, and lifestyle factors. Monitoring your response is essential when introducing new variables.

All combinations should be discussed with a qualified healthcare provider who understands both the pharmacokinetics of peptides and the interactions of nutritional compounds. Proper guidance ensures that dosing, timing, and interactions are optimized for your personal goals and physiology.

A well-planned peptide and nutrient strategy can create a synergistic effect, reinforcing the benefits of both while promoting overall resilience and healthspan.

Combining with Sleep, Hormone, or Anti-Aging Stacks

Strategically pairing peptides with other supplements can intensify their benefits across targeted goals like better sleep, hormonal equilibrium, and longevity support. When these substances are combined thoughtfully, they can reinforce one another's effects, creating a more comprehensive and effective approach to wellness.

Sleep optimization often begins with DSIP (Delta Sleep-Inducing Peptide), which promotes deeper, more restorative sleep phases. When stacked with supplements such as magnesium—known for its calming effects on the nervous system—or melatonin, which resets circadian rhythm timing, DSIP's impact can be magnified. Proper timing is essential; all components should align with your natural sleep-wake cycle for optimal effect.

For hormone balance, peptides like CJC-1295 and Ipamorelin support endogenous growth hormone release, which helps regulate metabolism, recovery, and body composition. These can be paired with zinc, which plays a role in testosterone metabolism, or vitamin D, which supports endocrine function. The result is a synergistic environment that promotes strength, energy, and hormonal stability.

Anti-aging stacks often include Epitalon, a peptide linked to telomere lengthening and cellular longevity. When used alongside antioxidants like resveratrol or glutathione, which counteract oxidative stress, and omega-3 fatty acids for cardiovascular and cognitive resilience, the anti-aging potential is expanded. This combination targets mitochondrial health, inflammation, and cellular regeneration.

To maximize results and minimize risk, supplement stacking should always be guided by an understanding of interactions, bioavailability, and timing. Some supplements may reduce peptide absorption or compete for metabolic pathways, while others can amplify the desired outcome.

This approach also requires individualization. Responses to peptides and supplements vary based on genetics, lifestyle, and existing nutrient status. Close observation and flexible adjustment are key to refining the stack.

Consulting with a knowledgeable healthcare provider ensures that combinations are tailored safely to your needs. With proper guidance, stacking peptides with targeted nutrients can create a cohesive system that elevates overall performance, recovery, and longevity.

Avoiding Counterproductive Interactions

When building an effective peptide and supplement regimen, avoiding negative interactions is just as important as selecting the right combinations. Stacking without careful consideration can reduce effectiveness or lead to unintended outcomes.

Certain nutrients may interfere with peptide absorption. Minerals like calcium and iron can bind to peptides in the digestive tract, limiting their uptake and diminishing their biological effect. To prevent this, these minerals should be taken several hours apart from peptide doses.

Supplemental actions may also contradict one another. Growth hormone-releasing peptides, for example, are often used for body recomposition and fat reduction. However, combining these with appetite-stimulating supplements—such as high-calorie mass gainers or certain forms of whey—could undermine fat loss goals by encouraging excess caloric intake.

Redundancy is another potential pitfall. Stacking multiple agents with the same mechanism of action— such as two or more growth hormone secretagogues or several stimulants—can lead to overstimulation, hormonal imbalance, or systemic stress. More is not always better; overlapping effects must be managed with precision.

Beyond supplements, lifestyle factors can significantly influence peptide efficacy. Alcohol, for instance, may impair liver function and interfere with peptide metabolism, reducing their effectiveness. Chronic sleep deprivation can blunt hormone sensitivity and weaken the natural rhythms many peptides are designed to support.

To minimize conflict and optimize synergy:

- Understand the mechanism of action of each peptide and supplement
- Avoid stacking items with overlapping or opposing effects without a clear purpose

- Separate timing for substances known to interfere with absorption
- Maintain awareness of how stress, sleep, and substance use may undermine results

Every stack should be approached with attention to detail and individualized adjustment. Biological responses vary based on genetics, health status, and lifestyle. Tracking personal feedback and fine-tuning accordingly is essential.

Professional oversight is highly recommended. A qualified healthcare provider can guide you in selecting compatible combinations, setting appropriate timing, and avoiding interactions that hinder results or introduce unnecessary risk.

Designing a successful peptide protocol isn't only about synergy—it's also about eliminating interference. A thoughtful approach ensures your regimen supports your goals without working against itself.

Timing Your Stack for Daily and Weekly Routines

Timing plays a central role in optimizing a peptide and supplement regimen. Aligning your protocol with natural biological rhythms and your weekly routine can enhance absorption, improve outcomes, and reduce the likelihood of interference.

Start by mapping out your daily schedule. Certain peptides yield greater benefits when timed to match the body's circadian patterns. Growth hormone-releasing peptides, for example, are generally most effective when taken in the evening, as the body's natural GH secretion peaks during deep sleep. In contrast, peptides or supplements aimed at boosting alertness, cognition, or physical performance are often better suited to morning use or pre-workout timing.

Meal timing is equally important. Some peptides, such as BPC-157, show higher bioavailability when taken on an empty stomach. Ingesting them away from meals reduces the risk of digestive enzymes breaking them down. On the other hand, certain fat-soluble vitamins and minerals require dietary fat for proper absorption and are best consumed with food.

Weekly structuring should reflect your activity cycles and recovery demands. If you're using peptides for muscle recovery, plan administration around your most intense training days to support tissue repair. Peptides that enhance sleep quality may benefit from a consistent nightly schedule, even on rest days, to reinforce a regular circadian rhythm.

Your cycling strategy also fits into this broader schedule. Periods of use followed by rest help prevent adaptation and sustain responsiveness. These cycles can be customized to support stressful phases, heavy training blocks, or recovery periods. For instance, incorporating a GH-releasing peptide during a strength-building phase, followed by a break during deload weeks, can help maintain long-term effectiveness.

Adaptability is key. Monitor your energy levels, sleep quality, recovery, and mental clarity to fine-tune the timing of each compound. Small adjustments to dosing windows can yield noticeable improvements.

Lastly, peptide and supplement protocols should be planned with guidance. A qualified healthcare provider can help align timing with your physiology and lifestyle demands, and offer ongoing support to refine your routine.

Strategic timing—daily and weekly—turns a collection of compounds into a cohesive, outcome-driven protocol. When built around your body's rhythms and needs, your stack becomes significantly more effective.

Tracking Progress for Optimization

Monitoring your body's response is essential for making a peptide regimen effective. Without consistent tracking, it's difficult to distinguish what's working from what's not—and impossible to make meaningful adjustments.

Tracking begins with clearly defined goals. Each peptide serves a specific purpose, and the metrics you choose should align with those objectives. For example:

- Muscle growth: monitor strength output, muscle mass, and body composition.
- Sleep improvement: track sleep duration, restfulness, and daytime energy levels.
- Cognitive performance or anti-aging: log mental clarity, mood stability, skin quality, or recovery time.

Data should be collected regularly and reviewed in context. Apps, journals, spreadsheets, or fitness trackers can all be effective tools. Whether you log morning energy, gym performance, or reaction time, the goal is to establish patterns that reflect how your protocol is performing.

Patterns often emerge gradually. A noticeable shift in sleep efficiency after introducing a nighttime peptide, or a consistent plateau in fat loss during a cycling break, can guide decisions on stacking, dosage, and timing.

Equally important is subjective feedback. Numbers matter, but so do energy levels, mood shifts, digestive changes, and overall vitality. Note how you feel after taking peptides, how you recover after workouts, or whether focus improves after cognitive support stacks. These subtle cues often precede measurable outcomes.

Adjustments should be based on trends—not isolated days. If a compound consistently produces noticeable benefit, consider adjusting the timing or dose. If results remain flat or regress, evaluate whether that peptide or supplement deserves a place in your stack.

Work closely with a qualified healthcare provider throughout. They can help interpret data, make evidence-based adjustments, and ensure your regimen remains effective and safe.

Tracking is not simply a log of progress—it's a roadmap for continuous refinement. When approached with consistency and attention, it becomes one of the most powerful tools in any peptide strategy.

CHAPTER 11

COMMON MISTAKES AND HOW TO AVOID THEM

Overdosing and Overlapping Peptides

Peptides are powerful tools, but their misuse—especially through overdosing and poorly planned overlaps—can lead to diminished benefits and potential health risks. Proper dosage and stack design are critical to safety and effectiveness.

Overdosing occurs when peptide quantities exceed recommended thresholds. This often results in overstimulation of targeted biological processes. For growth hormone-releasing peptides (GHRPs), excessive dosing can trigger side effects such as bloating, joint stiffness, numbness, insulin resistance, or even elevated cardiovascular risk. Symptoms like these signal an imbalance that may require immediate adjustment.

Overlapping peptides—using multiple compounds with similar effects—can compound these problems. While stacking can create synergy, overlapping too many peptides with the same mechanism (e.g., multiple GHRPs or multiple cognitive enhancers) can overload receptors, desensitize pathways, and blunt overall progress. This disrupts the body's feedback systems and often results in paradoxical fatigue, irritability, or hormonal dysregulation.

To prevent these outcomes:

- Understand each peptide's mechanism. Avoid combining compounds that compete for the same pathway or amplify the same effect.
- Respect clinical dose ranges. More is not better. Use the minimum effective dose and titrate only if needed.

- Avoid redundant stacking. If two peptides target the same hormone or neurotransmitter, consider using only one or alternating them.
- Cycle regularly. Periods of rest prevent receptor fatigue and support long-term responsiveness.

Personal tolerance, existing hormone levels, age, and metabolic health all influence how peptides are processed. Begin with a single compound to assess tolerance and response before adding others. Stagger introduction timelines when expanding your stack.

Tracking symptoms and outcomes is key. Unusual side effects, fatigue, swelling, sleep disruption, or mood changes may indicate overstimulation or imbalance. Adjust or pause use accordingly.

Finally, consult with a healthcare provider who understands advanced peptide use. A professional can ensure that your stack is both safe and optimized for your goals.

Avoiding dosing mistakes and inappropriate overlaps isn't just about avoiding setbacks—it's how you build a protocol that delivers results over time without taxing your system.

Ignoring Side Effects or Overusing Stimulatory Peptides

One of the most overlooked yet impactful mistakes in peptide use is failing to respond to side effects or relying too heavily on stimulatory compounds. Both can disrupt physiological balance and limit long-term results.

Peptides, like any biologically active agent, can produce adverse effects. These may be mild—such as localized irritation at injection sites—or systemic, such as fatigue, swelling, appetite changes, or hormone dysregulation. Dismissing these signs as minor or pushing through discomfort undermines both safety and effectiveness. Early symptoms often serve as a warning that dosage or peptide selection may need adjustment.

For instance, users of growth hormone-releasing peptides frequently report joint stiffness, fluid retention, or numbness in extremities. These are not rare responses—they are physiological cues requiring attention. Similarly, peptides affecting neurotransmitters may cause overstimulation, resulting in jitteriness, anxiety, or insomnia.

Another common misstep is overreliance on stimulatory peptides. Compounds like CJC-1295, Ipamorelin, or nootropics such as Semax and Noopept can offer sharp benefits for performance and cognitive clarity—but frequent or high-dose use can overwhelm the body's regulatory systems. Long-term overstimulation risks desensitizing receptors or elevating certain hormones to unsafe levels.

Growth hormone excess, for example, can lead to tissue swelling, disrupted glucose metabolism, or in extreme cases, features of acromegaly. On the neurological side, constant stimulation from cognitive peptides may worsen mood instability, sleep disorders, or induce mental fatigue.

Best practices to avoid these outcomes include:

- Monitor symptoms closely. Any recurring or worsening effects are signals to pause, reassess, or lower your dose.
- Use the lowest effective dose. Increase only when clearly beneficial and well tolerated.
- Cycle off regularly. Give your system time to recalibrate and avoid receptor desensitization.
- Prioritize foundational health. No peptide can replace the benefits of proper nutrition, sleep, and recovery.

Subjective feedback matters. Energy fluctuations, disrupted sleep, mood shifts, or appetite changes can all reflect overstimulation or imbalance. Keep a log to identify patterns and share it with your provider during follow-ups.

Most importantly, avoid assuming that more is better. The precision of peptides lies in their targeted activity—effective use demands equally precise dosing and timing. Consult a knowledgeable practitioner to guide peptide selection, duration, and responsiveness based on your profile.

Used correctly, peptides can accelerate progress. Used recklessly, they can derail it. Responsible use, thoughtful tracking, and a balanced protocol form the foundation of a successful regimen.

Not Supporting Recovery or Nutrition Properly

A frequent yet critical oversight in peptide use is the failure to support recovery and nutrition. Peptides can accelerate healing, growth, and performance—but without proper rest and dietary support, their potential is significantly diminished.

Recovery is a biological necessity. Peptides that promote muscle repair or aid in tissue regeneration rely on the body's innate healing cycles, particularly those triggered during deep sleep. For example, peptides that stimulate growth hormone release are most effective when paired with quality sleep, as growth hormone is secreted predominantly during slow-wave sleep. Disrupted rest undermines both peptide function and the benefits they're designed to support.

Physical overexertion without adequate rest blunts the regenerative effects of peptides and increases susceptibility to inflammation, injury, and hormonal dysregulation. Even peptides with anti-inflammatory or healing properties cannot offset the physiological cost of chronic overtraining.

Nutrition is equally foundational. Peptides do not build tissue, balance hormones, or optimize metabolic function in isolation—they support processes that rely on macro- and micronutrients. A peptide targeting muscle growth, for instance, requires an adequate protein intake to supply the amino acids needed for hypertrophy. A calorie deficit can impede anabolic signaling, even in the presence of peptide-induced growth hormone release.

Micronutrients also play an amplifying role. For instance:

- Vitamin C supports collagen synthesis, enhancing the effects of peptides like GHK-Cu or BPC-157.
- Zinc and magnesium contribute to hormonal balance, benefiting users of hormone-modulating peptides.
- Omega-3 fatty acids reduce inflammation and complement healing peptides during recovery.

Without sufficient dietary input, the biochemical actions initiated by peptides remain incomplete.

To avoid this pitfall:

- Prioritize 7–9 hours of uninterrupted, quality sleep.
- Maintain protein intake at levels appropriate for your goals (typically 0.7–1g per pound of lean body mass for most active individuals).
- Ensure your diet includes nutrient-dense whole foods and limits processed, inflammatory inputs.
- Time rest days and recovery-focused peptides strategically after high-stress physical exertion.

Peptides are catalysts—they work best in systems that are already supported. They cannot replace the basics of biological repair.

Work with a healthcare provider or nutritionist to align your peptide use with evidence-based recovery and nutrition strategies. Adjust both training and dietary protocols alongside your supplementation for optimal synergy.

Failing to support recovery and nutrition is not just inefficient—it risks blunting the long-term potential of your peptide regimen. A well-fed, well-rested body is the most effective environment for peptides to exert their intended benefits.

Misunderstanding Labels and Protocols

One of the most overlooked yet consequential errors in peptide use is misinterpreting labels and misunderstanding protocols. Peptides are precise biological tools, and even minor missteps in how they're handled, dosed, or stored can compromise their effects or introduce avoidable risks.

Labels often display concentration in milligrams (mg), but peptide dosages are typically administered in micrograms (mcg). Misreading this distinction can result in a dose ten times higher—or lower—than intended. For example, a 5mg vial may need to be diluted in 2mL of bacteriostatic water. To administer a 500mcg dose from this solution, you'd need to measure exactly 0.2mL using a calibrated syringe. An incorrect interpretation of the label could lead to over- or underdosing, both of which reduce effectiveness and increase risk.

Protocols also vary widely. Some peptides require administration on an empty stomach to avoid enzymatic breakdown, while others benefit from co-ingestion with food. Timing matters, too—growth hormone secretagogues like Ipamorelin or CJC-1295 are most effective when taken at night, syncing with the body's natural hormone rhythm. In contrast, nootropic peptides may perform better earlier in the day.

Storage errors are another common issue. Most peptides must be refrigerated after reconstitution, and some require freezing prior to mixing. Room temperature storage may cause degradation, reducing both potency and shelf life. Labels often include specific instructions, but users unfamiliar with peptide chemistry may ignore or misapply them.

To avoid these pitfalls:

- Read labels carefully. Understand the difference between mg and mcg, and calculate dosages accordingly.
- Dilute with precision. Use bacteriostatic water, sterile vials, and insulin syringes for accurate measurement.
- Follow administration timing. Align peptide timing with digestion, sleep, or activity cycles as recommended for each compound.
- Store properly. Keep peptides in a clean, cold, and dark environment. Reconstituted solutions should be refrigerated, and dry powder should be kept sealed and temperature-controlled.

If any step is unclear, consult a pharmacist, healthcare provider, or experienced practitioner. Improvising or guessing with peptides undermines their reliability and safety.

Understanding peptide labels and protocols is not optional—it is foundational. Missteps in measurement, timing, or storage create compounding errors that diminish the benefits of your protocol. A meticulous approach ensures you extract the full value from each compound and protect your health throughout the process.

Building a Smart, Sustainable Strategy

The foundation of effective peptide use lies in creating a strategy that is both intelligent and sustainable. Rather than relying on shortcuts or chasing rapid transformation, a thoughtful approach helps ensure long-term results and minimizes the risks often associated with misuse.

A well-designed peptide regimen begins with specific, clearly defined goals. Whether you're focused on building lean muscle, accelerating fat loss, improving sleep, enhancing cognitive clarity, or supporting anti-aging processes, your objectives shape every aspect of your protocol—from compound selection to timing and delivery method.

Equally important is the understanding that peptides cannot compensate for poor lifestyle habits. These compounds function best as part of a broader, integrated wellness plan. Solid nutrition, consistent exercise, high-quality sleep, and daily stress reduction are not optional—they are prerequisites. Peptides amplify progress, but they cannot generate it in the absence of foundational health practices.

Long-term success also requires patience and responsibility. Avoid jumping into high doses or stacking multiple peptides without a clear rationale. Begin conservatively, allowing time to evaluate your body's response before increasing frequency or dosage. Use cycling protocols to avoid receptor desensitization, overreliance, or systemic fatigue.

Sustainability also means flexibility. Monitor your body's signals and adjust accordingly. Recovery needs, metabolic rate, hormonal shifts, and stress levels can fluctuate over time, and your strategy must adapt to meet those evolving demands.

A smart protocol is one that can be realistically maintained—not just for weeks, but for months and years. Overcomplicating your regimen with unnecessary compounds, imprecise dosing, or erratic timing creates more risk than reward. Simple, well-aligned strategies are far more effective and manageable.

Guidance from a knowledgeable healthcare provider is essential. Professional input ensures proper dosing, guards against adverse interactions, and offers a framework for periodic reassessment. Peptides are highly targeted tools, and their use benefits from professional insight and oversight.

Building a sustainable peptide strategy means setting measurable goals, supporting your protocol with healthy habits, using peptides with precision, and refining your regimen over time. This deliberate, well-balanced approach not only protects your health but helps unlock the full therapeutic potential of peptides in a safe and dependable way.

CHAPTER 12

THE FUTURE OF PEPTIDE BIOHACKING

Cutting-Edge Peptides Entering the Market

Peptide research is advancing rapidly, ushering in a new generation of precision compounds aimed at optimizing human performance, longevity, and cognitive function. These novel peptides are the product of sophisticated bioengineering and clinical insight, offering enhanced specificity, improved targeting, and broader applications than their predecessors.

Unlike earlier compounds with broad systemic effects, these next-generation peptides are designed to interact with narrowly defined biological pathways. This specificity reduces the risk of unwanted side effects while amplifying their therapeutic potential. Emerging peptides are not only more refined in action but also reflect a deeper understanding of genetic signaling, cellular repair mechanisms, and age-related decline.

Several investigational peptides are targeting mechanisms directly tied to aging. By modulating the expression of genes associated with cellular senescence and mitochondrial function, these compounds are showing potential in delaying degenerative changes and supporting systemic rejuvenation. While still under study, their ability to influence longevity markers has generated significant interest in both clinical and self-optimization circles.

Cognitive enhancement is another area seeing groundbreaking developments. Peptides are being formulated to target neurotrophic factors, synaptic density, and neurotransmitter regulation. These compounds are being studied for their capacity to enhance memory consolidation, sharpen focus, and promote neuroprotection—applications that extend from age-related cognitive decline to high-performance mental output.

In athletic performance, a new class of peptides is emerging with the aim of supporting muscle regeneration, boosting ATP production, and accelerating recovery without triggering the hormonal disruption or side effects seen in anabolic agents. These developments may offer athletes and fitness enthusiasts a safer, biologically compatible option for performance support.

Examples of novel compounds include mitochondrial-targeted peptides that improve cellular energy efficiency, senolytic peptides that selectively clear senescent cells, and gene-regulatory peptides designed to influence circadian rhythm and DNA repair. These innovations reflect a shift from symptomatic treatment to root-level intervention.

While many of these peptides are still under evaluation in preclinical or early-phase human trials, their arrival signals a major evolution in how we approach personalized wellness, therapeutic prevention, and regenerative care. Regulatory scrutiny remains high, and access to some of these peptides may be restricted pending broader safety validation.

Still, the trajectory is clear: peptide biohacking is moving toward smarter, more individualized protocols that combine data-driven precision with biological nuance. These compounds are not replacements for foundational health practices, but they represent a powerful extension of what's possible when science meets self-care.

As with any advancement in therapeutic technology, careful implementation is essential. These peptides must be approached with a solid understanding of mechanism, risk, and context—ideally under professional supervision. Used correctly, they may redefine what it means to maintain vitality, enhance function, and age with intention.

Where the Research Is Headed

The landscape of peptide research is expanding rapidly, fueled by innovation in biotechnology and a growing interest in personalized health solutions. Scientists worldwide are uncovering new applications for peptides that extend far beyond traditional supplementation, pushing the boundaries of what is possible in regenerative medicine, precision therapy, and preventative care.

One of the most compelling directions involves individualized peptide protocols. By leveraging genetic, metabolic, and lifestyle data, researchers aim to design peptide treatments tailored to a person's unique biology. This approach could significantly improve outcomes by ensuring precise targeting and minimizing non-responsiveness or side effects.

In parallel, peptides are being explored as agents of precision medicine—interventions that act on specific molecular pathways tied to chronic disease. These compounds offer the advantage of selectivity, capable of influencing key cellular signals without disrupting surrounding physiological processes. This positions peptides as potential tools in managing complex diseases with higher efficacy and fewer adverse reactions.

Regenerative medicine is another frontier drawing heavy research investment. Certain peptides, such as BPC-157 and TB-500, show promise in promoting angiogenesis, collagen synthesis, and tissue repair. These properties are under investigation for applications ranging from gastrointestinal recovery to tendon healing and joint regeneration.

Neurobiology is also a focus, particularly the use of peptides to enhance brain resilience and function. Several compounds under study have demonstrated the ability to protect neurons, improve synaptic plasticity, and support neurochemical balance. Their potential roles in delaying cognitive decline and supporting treatment-resistant neurological disorders are being closely examined.

Anti-aging science is rapidly integrating peptide research. Investigators are examining compounds that influence telomere length, mitochondrial function, and DNA repair. Some peptides, like Epitalon, have already shown effects on longevity-related markers in early studies, prompting deeper investigation into their role in extending healthspan.

In addition to expanding applications, researchers are developing delivery systems that increase peptide bioavailability and stability. Techniques such as nanoencapsulation, transdermal patches, and oral delivery innovations are opening new routes for administration without compromising efficacy.

While enthusiasm is warranted, the field remains in early stages. Most peptides are still undergoing clinical evaluation or remain experimental. Long-term effects, ideal dosing strategies, and full safety profiles require further validation before broad adoption.

A cautious and informed approach remains essential. Peptides should complement—not replace—core wellness strategies like nutrition, movement, sleep, and emotional regulation. Used wisely, they hold potential to become foundational tools in the future of integrated, proactive healthcare.

Personalized Peptide Stacks with AI and Lab Testing

Peptide biohacking is evolving beyond broad-spectrum approaches. The future lies in personalization—fine-tuned regimens built around individual biology. Personalized peptide stacks, powered by artificial intelligence and informed by lab diagnostics, represent the next frontier in precision health optimization.

A personalized peptide stack is a curated combination of peptides selected according to an individual's unique physiological profile and health objectives. Rather than applying generic protocols, this strategy tailors interventions to the individual—taking into account genetics, biomarkers, lifestyle, and specific goals.

This process begins with comprehensive lab testing. Blood panels, hormone profiles, micronutrient assessments, and inflammatory markers offer critical data points. These insights reveal functional imbalances, deficiencies, or overactive pathways—each of which can be addressed with the appropriate peptide compound.

AI plays a pivotal role by processing and interpreting this complex dataset. It identifies patterns and correlations that might be missed through manual analysis, offering peptide recommendations that match the individual's current biological state. Age, sex, metabolic status, stress response, sleep quality, and existing medical conditions are all factored into the algorithm's recommendation engine.

For example:

- Low IGF-1 levels and disrupted circadian markers might lead to a recommendation of CJC-1295 and DSIP.
- Elevated systemic inflammation and gut permeability might call for a stack including BPC-157 and Thymosin Beta-4.
- Suboptimal testosterone and high cortisol could guide the inclusion of Kisspeptin-10 alongside adaptogenic support.

This integration of AI and lab results allows for unmatched precision—selecting the right peptides, in the right order, at the right dosage, with consideration for synergistic interactions and cycling schedules.

Yet, while AI provides data-driven recommendations, clinical oversight remains essential. Algorithms lack the intuition and context a seasoned healthcare practitioner provides. Interpretations should be validated by a professional who can adjust protocols in real time and provide human-centered decision-making.

It's also important to remember that lab results represent snapshots, not final answers. Biological markers change with diet, stress, environment, and time. Periodic retesting is essential to track outcomes and recalibrate protocols.

Building and refining a personalized peptide stack is an ongoing process—iterative, responsive, and dynamic. As new peptides are developed and more data becomes available, these stacks can evolve to better match changing physiological needs and life phases.

The convergence of AI technology, biomarker testing, and peptide science holds the potential to redefine preventive and performance-based medicine. It represents a shift from reactive health management to proactive, personalized optimization.

By leveraging data intelligently and integrating peptide science within a broader wellness framework, individuals can achieve measurable, sustainable progress in health, performance, and longevity.

Ethical, Legal, and Accessibility Issues

The future of peptide biohacking brings immense potential—but also raises pressing ethical, legal, and accessibility concerns. These issues are critical in determining how peptides will be integrated responsibly into health systems, wellness strategies, and society at large.

Ethically, peptides challenge long-standing norms in performance, enhancement, and equity. In competitive sports, the use of peptides for physical or cognitive enhancement poses dilemmas around fairness. Should access to biologically augmenting compounds be regulated in competition? What separates enhancement from treatment? These questions have no simple answers and will require ongoing dialogue between regulators, ethicists, and the public.

There are also broader equity concerns. When only a subset of the population can afford or access cutting-edge peptide therapies, disparities in health and performance outcomes may widen. Without frameworks that ensure responsible access, peptide biohacking risks becoming a tool that amplifies privilege rather than supporting broad wellness.

Legally, the peptide landscape is inconsistent and often opaque. In the U.S., many peptides remain unapproved by the FDA for human use and are sold under the label of "research chemicals." While this allows access, it also opens the door to poorly regulated sources, inconsistent quality, and risks to user safety.

Other countries impose stricter regulations, making even medically supervised access difficult. This inconsistency creates a fragmented global market, where legality depends more on jurisdiction than on scientific consensus or therapeutic value.

Accessibility poses another significant barrier. Peptides can be prohibitively expensive, especially when used in long-term protocols. Most are not covered by insurance. Add to this the complexity of use—reconstitution, sterile handling, dose timing, and cycling—and it becomes clear that peptide biohacking remains inaccessible to many.

Solutions may involve the development of simplified delivery methods, improved education, and regulatory clarity. If peptides are to become a tool for public health—not just elite optimization—they must be easier to access, afford, and understand.

There is also an urgent need for medical literacy. Patients and consumers need clear, evidence-based resources. Healthcare providers must be educated on peptide science so they can provide accurate guidance. Without widespread understanding, misinformation can flourish, increasing the likelihood of misuse or harm.

These challenges are not insurmountable. As scientific support for peptides grows, regulatory frameworks may adapt to reflect legitimate medical uses. Ethics committees and insurers may evolve policies that distinguish therapeutic from enhancement use. Accessibility could be improved through education, subsidization, or simplified over-the-counter options where appropriate.

For the field of peptide biohacking to mature responsibly, it must address these structural and societal issues head-on—not as an afterthought, but as a core part of its development. Innovation without responsibility creates fragility, not progress.

A future where peptides are safe, ethical, legal, and accessible is possible—but only with foresight, cooperation, and commitment to equity.

Final Thoughts on Responsible, Informed Use

As we close this comprehensive journey into the world of peptides, one truth becomes clear: these compounds offer extraordinary potential, but only when approached with responsibility and understanding. Peptides are not shortcuts—they are tools, and how we use them determines their value.

Responsible use begins with restraint. Start low. Titrate slowly. Observe how your body responds before making adjustments. Cycling protocols should include rest phases to prevent desensitization and hormonal disruption. This is not about chasing extremes—it's about long-term optimization.

Equally vital is the context in which peptides are used. No protocol exists in isolation. Diet, sleep, training, stress levels, and overall lifestyle determine how effective peptides will be. Skipping these fundamentals while relying solely on biochemical enhancement is a recipe for imbalance. Peptides amplify good habits—they don't replace them.

Informed use demands education. Know what you're using. Understand its mechanism, benefits, limitations, and possible side effects. Stay current with emerging science. Engage critically with sources. And above all, seek expert medical guidance. Even the most advanced stack means little if applied blindly or recklessly.

Ethical and legal awareness is also essential. Many peptides occupy regulatory gray zones—some are research-use only, while others are legally prescribed. Know your local laws. Use discretion. Advocate for responsible frameworks, not deregulated chaos. Biohacking should be a movement toward empowerment, not exploitation.

Finally, accessibility must be part of the conversation. Cost, complexity, and limited clinical adoption create barriers. Broader access—when rooted in safety and education—benefits not just individuals but public health. Advocacy means working toward a future where evidence-based peptide protocols are available to all who need them, not just the elite few.

Peptides hold remarkable potential. But they are not magic. They are not replacements for fundamentals. They are not immune to misuse. A responsible, informed approach ensures that their promise doesn't become a pitfall.

The future of biohacking lies not in reckless experimentation, but in thoughtful application. Use peptides as part of a deliberate, data-driven strategy—guided by curiosity, grounded in science, and committed to health over hype.

That is the path forward. That is how we unlock the true potential of peptide therapeutics.

CONCLUSION

This journey into the science, application, and promise of peptides has covered a vast landscape—from foundational biology to cutting-edge protocols. As we close this chapter, the takeaway is clear: peptides offer tremendous potential, but only for those willing to approach them with intention, structure, and long-term thinking.

Peptides are more than biochemical tools—they are programmable molecules with targeted capabilities. Their effects range from stimulating growth hormone, improving fat metabolism, enhancing sleep, supporting recovery, to optimizing neurological performance. Each one interacts with the body through specific pathways, offering a level of precision rarely found in traditional supplements.

Designing a protocol is about aligning intervention with intent. Selection should reflect your current physiology and your long-term objectives. Start with clearly defined goals. Choose peptides with complementary actions. Apply informed dosing and cycle intentionally. Stack with synergy—not complexity. Track what matters. Adjust as needed.

Begin with simplicity. Use one peptide. Low dose. One variable at a time. Create a baseline with measurable data: sleep logs, strength metrics, mood journals, cognitive scores. Refine from there. Personalization is not a feature—it is the foundation.

Your needs will shift. That's inevitable. Peptides can evolve with you. A phase focused on recovery might later pivot to cognitive support. What works at 35 might differ at 55. Adapt your protocol as your biology, goals, and environment change. Stay current with research. Seek feedback from qualified professionals. Make data your ally.

Avoid shortcuts. Peptides can amplify, but they do not replace:

- Quality sleep
- Nutrient-dense food

- Daily movement
- Stress regulation
- Purpose-driven living

All peptide strategies are downstream from these fundamentals.

The future of peptide use is personalized, data-driven, and increasingly democratized. With lab testing, AI, and emerging delivery systems, the potential is growing—but so is the need for discernment. Stay curious. Stay cautious. Stay grounded.

This book was written to empower—not just with knowledge, but with strategy. You now have a foundation. Use it to build something sustainable. Something smart. Something that serves your health now and in decades to come.

Peptides are not the journey. They are companions along the way.

Here's to a future of clarity, strength, and resilience. The next steps are yours.

Stay deliberate. Stay informed. Stay vital.

Made in United States
Orlando, FL
23 July 2025

63193681R00052